Techniques of Regional Anaesthesia

Techniques of Regional Anaesthesia

D. BRUCE SCOTT
M.D., F.R.C.P.E., F.F.A.R.C.S.

Consultant Anaesthetist,
Royal Infirmary; and
Senior Lecturer,
Department of Anaesthetics,
University of Edinburgh,
Edinburgh, Scotland

LENNART HÅKANSSON
Coordinator

POUL BUCKHÖJ
Medical artist

Foreword by
PHILLIP R. BROMAGE
M.B., B.S., F.F.A.R.C.S., FRCP(C)

APPLETON & LANGE/MEDIGLOBE
Norwalk, Connecticut/San Mateo, California/Fribourg, Switzerland

Notice: Our knowledge in clinical sciences is constantly changing. As new information becomes available, changes in treatment and in the use of drugs become necessary. The author(s) and the publisher of this volume have taken care to make certain that the doses of drugs and schedules of treatment are correct and compatible with the standards generally accepted at the time of publication. The reader is advised to consult carefully the instruction and information material included in the package insert of each drug or therapeutic agent before administration. This advice is especially important when using new or infrequently used drugs.

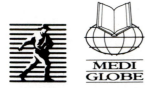

MEDI GLOBE

Copyright © 1989 Mediglobe S.A.
(ISBN 2-88239-009-2)
Published throughout the world in English by Appleton & Lange - a Publishing Division of Prentice Hall - in conjunction with Mediglobe S.A.

89 90 91 / 10 9 8 7 6 5 4 3 2 1

Prentice-Hall of Australia, Pty.Ltd., Sydney
Prentice-Hall Canada, Inc.
Prentice-Hall Hispanoamericana, S.A., Mexico
Prentice-Hall or India Private Limited, New Delhi
Prentice-Hall of Japan, Inc., Tokyo
Prentice-Hall of Southeast Asia (Pte.) Ltd., Singapore
Whitehall Books Ltd., Wellington, New Zealand
Editora Prentice-Hall do Brasil Ltda., Rio de Janeiro

Printed by
KIN KEONG PRINTING PTE LTD
SINGAPORE

Library of Congress Cataloging-in-Publication Data

Scott, D. Bruce (Donald Bruce)
    Techniques of regional anesthesia.

Includes index.
1. Conduction anesthesia--Handbooks, manuals, etc.
I. Title. (DNLM: 1. Anesthesia, Conduction-methods. WO 300 S425t)
RD84.S472 1989
617'.964   88-10373

ISBN 0-8385-8844-1

Foreword

Regional anaesthesia has undergone a renaissance of interest and widening clinical applications during the past three decades. Skill in the art of regional anaesthesia does not come easily to all students. As a craft it needs the interactions of master craftsmen and dedicated apprentices. Expertise, gentleness and an inward eye for hidden anatomical structures are the prerequisites for safety and success.

Specialty texts abound, but the tyro needs an easy-to-read, bird's eye view of the subject, combined with an intuitive focus to bring him under the patient's skin, into the hidden three-dimensional world of living anatomy that only the needle-tip sees. He needs this with just enough text to give him basic essentials of supporting theory, without distracting him from his practical task by excessive emphasis on theoretical details. They can come later.

This book is worthy successor to the Illustrated Handbook of Local Anaesthesia (1969) that was the product of collaboration between the present artist, Poul Buckhöj and Dr. Ejnar Eriksson, and it combines the insights of a master craftsman-teacher in regional anaesthesia with those of a master artist in medical illustration. Between them they have created a series of visual and mental images that cover the whole field of regional anaesthesia with remarkabale clarity and conviction, and their work is the practical answer to the student's question "What should I read?" It is also the answer to the single-handed practitioner in remote places, where the luminous pictures and the crisp text can give him the assurance and precise anatomical guidance that he needs when working alone.

Techniques of Regional Anaesthesia will be warmly welcomed by trainees and teachers alike as easy to read and as a clear and accurate guide to successful techniques.

Philip R. Bromage,
M.B., B.S., F.F.A.R.C.S., FRCP (C)
Professor of Anaesthesia
King Khalid University Hospital
Riyadh
The Kingdom of Saudi Arabia

Preface

Writing and publishing a comprehensive volume of regional anaesthetic techniques, when several similar books are already available, needs some explanation.

Those who work in the field will be familiar with the Illustrated Handbook in Local Anaesthesia edited by Ejnar Eriksson, first published in 1969, the last edition appearing in 1979. This very popular book stood out from the rest by virtue of the excellence of its coloured figures, particularly the anatomical drawings by Poul Buckhöj.

However, no discipline in medicine stands still. It became apparent that to provide an up to date text, and to include as many techniques relevant to modern practice as possible, a new book was required.

Regional anaesthesia serves three main areas, surgical anaesthesia, obstetric analgesia, and pain relief. The principles behind the application of regional anaesthesia often differ considerably between these three indications, but the actual techniques are largely the same and, of course, the anatomy does not alter.

The background to regional anaesthesia, including the pharmacology of local anaesthetics, the management of patients and the treatment of complications, is given in the introduction. Thereafter the techniques are described according to the region of the body. Finally a chapter on postoperative pain relief using regional anaesthetic techniques has been added.

We have been allowed to use drawings and photoes from other productions from the same publisher, MEDIGLOBE, and we are grateful to the authors of:
Illustrated Handbook of Local Anaesthesia, E. Eriksson
Handbook of Dental Local Anaesthesia, H. Evers, G. Haegerstam
Plexus Anesthesia I, Perivascular Techniques of Brachial Plexus Block, A.P. Winnie
Atlas of Cystoscopy, J. Schönebeck
Handbook of Epidural Anaesthesia and Analgesia B.G. Covino, D.R. Scott
Handbook of Thoraco-abdominal Nerve Block, J. Katz, H. Renck

Fortunately we have been able to retain the services of Poul Buckhöj, who has made many new drawings.

Drug nomenclature follows the World Health Organisation's International Non-proprietary Name (INN) convention. Gray's Anatomy (35th ed, editors R. Warwick and P.L. Williams) has been our main reference for anatomy.

It must surely cross the reader's mind that no one practitioner could be proficient in, or even have a passing familiarity with, all the techniques included. In deciding on single rather than multi authorship, it was felt that this would give, for better or worse, a consistent style. Where the author's personal experience was lacking, he took advice from experts and can vouch for the practicality of the methods described in the book. I suspect that many an editor of multi-author books will feel a pang of envy at one who could make his own decisions reasonably quickly. To those who have helped me, colleagues in Edinburgh and many other friends worldwide, too many indeed to name individually, go my heartfelt thanks. I have picked their brains unmercifully, but I hope to good effect. Those from whom I begged, borrowed or almost stole radiographs, have been acknowledged in the text. If this book has any success, it is due to Poul Buckhöj for the beautiful drawings, Lennart Håkansson as co-ordinator and layout artist, Tom McFetters and Karsten Hjertholm who took the photographs, and Pam Hindshaw, my secretary.

D. Bruce Scott

7

Contents

Introduction

Use of local or regional anaesthesia

Local or regional anaesthesia may be used for surgical procedures, for relief of acute or chronic pain, and for therapeutic or diagnostic purposes.

Advantages

The ability to render a specific part of the body anaesthetic without affecting the brain has many advantages, including:

1. The ability to have the patient conscious during surgery. Thus the patient can maintain his own airway and the inhalation of gastric contents is unlikely. For minor procedures, the presence of an anaesthetist is unnecessary.

2. A smooth recovery. Unlike general anaesthesia, many procedures do not require the same degree of nursing care that is necessary with an unconscious patient. Because in most cases local anaesthesia will still be present at the end of surgery, the patient will be awake and rational when pain eventually appears. This contrasts with the restlessness frequently seen in the semiconscious patient with severe pain after general anaesthesia.

3. Postoperative analgesia. In many instances it is possible to continue the local anaesthesia for hours or days, e.g. by using a catheter technique.

4. Reduction in surgical stress. The elimination of painful afferent stimuli from the operative site, plus the blockade of efferent sympathetic nerves to endocrine glands, eliminates or greatly reduces the metabolic and endocrine changes seen after surgical operations. This applies in the main to lower abdominal, perineal and limb surgery. The modification of surgical stress will be greatest when the local anaesthesia is continued for 1-2 days postoperatively.

5. Earlier discharge for outpatients or day patients.

6. Less expense.

Disadvantages

1. The patient may prefer to be asleep. This does not preclude the use of regional anaesthesia, which can be combined with a light general anaesthetic.

2. A degree of practice and skill is required for the best results. Operations on awake patients also involve the cooperation of the whole surgical team.

3. Some blocks require up to 30 min or more to be fully effective.

4. Analgesia may not always be totally effective. Thus the patient may require additional analgesics, or a light general anaesthetic.

5. Generalised toxicity may occur if the local anaesthetic drug is given intravenously by mistake, or an overdose is injected.

6. Some operations, e.g. thoracotomies, are unsuitable for local anaesthesia.

7. Widespread sympathetic blockade with resulting hypotension can occur with certain techniques, e.g. spinal or epidural blockade.

8. There is a small but definite incidence of prolonged nerve damage.

Preoperative assessment and preparation

The preoperative assessment of patients is not different from that required for general anaesthesia. Thus it is necessary to determine the general physical condition, to identify any relevant pathology and to assess the patient's attitude to the proposed anaesthetic technique.

The need to perform surgery using local or regional anaesthesia may vary from "mandatory" to "contraindicated" depending on circumstances. Thus a patient with an airway which cannot be guaranteed during general anaesthesia and who may be at risk from inhalation of gastric contents, requires to be awake during surgery. A patient with a strong desire to be awake, e.g. for the performance of a Caesarean section, will consider regional anaesthesia highly desirable. In other patients, widespread sympathetic blockade may be an unacceptable risk, e.g. those with uncorrected hypovolaemia.

Many patients may be unwilling at first to accept a local/regional anaesthetic. However, a proper explanation of the risks and the benefits will usually prevail if the indication is well based. The possibility of performing the operation using a combination of regional and general anaesthesia should also be considered. Indeed, this often provides the best anaesthesia for the patient. Only in exceptional cases should a patient be obliged to remain awake, if they have strong objections.

Premedication

This will depend upon the individual patient, whether or not he or she will remain conscious, and on the anaesthetist's preference. No premedicant drugs are contraindicated in regional anaesthesia.

Management during anaesthesia and surgery

During the preparation for, and the performance of, the local/regional anaesthesia, the way in which the patient is treated is of great importance. An accurate explanation of what is to happen step by step, will get the patient's confidence. If a concomitant general anaesthetic is planned, there is a temptation to put the patient "to sleep" before performing the local technique. This may indeed be desirable, e.g. in a child, but many techniques are better done with the patient conscious so as to assess such things as paraesthesia or accidental intravenous injection, before any general anaesthesia is given.

In all but the most trivial procedures, no local anaesthetic drug should be injected unless all the necessary apparatus (including that needed for monitoring) and drugs which may be required for resuscitation are at hand. In general these will be identical to those required for other types of anaesthesia.

Intravenous access is particularly important and should be ensured by an indwelling needle or IV infusion before the regional technique is performed.

The injection of local anaesthetic drug is of course the **start** and not the **end** of the anaesthesia. Once the block has been performed, the management will depend upon whether or not the patient is to remain awake or be rendered unconscious with a light general anaesthetic.

Conscious patients

Conscious patients will require special management which should include:

1. Delaying the operation and its preparation until the local anaesthetic has produced its full effect. Impatience in this respect is one of the commonest reasons for failure of regional anaesthesia.

2. Ensuring that **all** members of the surgical team are aware that the patient is conscious. Loud noises and injudicious conversation can greatly alarm patients who are usually quite unused to the operation room environment. Nurses, doctors and attendants should be calm, solicitous and considerate towards the patient.

3. The patient should be made comfortable on the operating table.

4. The patient should be reassured that the anaesthetist is always immediately available and able to deal with any problems.

5. If there is a complaint of pain or discomfort, the anaesthetist should explain the reason and treat it as indicated. It is never a good idea to tell the patient beforehand that he/she "will feel nothing". This is frequently untrue and the patient will lose confidence. Most patients will tolerate some discomfort if it is short-lived, e.g. during delivery of the baby's head at Caesarean section. If there is a deficiency in the effectiveness of the block, then an analgesic drug, preferably an opioid, should be given intravenously, e.g. morphine 10 mg, diamorphine 5 mg, pethidine 100 mg or fentanyl 100 μg. Do not treat pain initially with a sedative or tranquillising drug. These have no analgesic properties and frequently cause the patient to become irrational and uncooperative. The sedative properties of opioids are usually sufficient once they have controlled the pain.

6. If, in the absence of pain, the patient becomes frightened or hysterical, a tranquilliser such as diazepam 5-10 mg given slowly IV may become necessary. Remember that irrational and hysterical behaviour may be evidence of generalised toxicity to the local anaesthetic drug.

7. It may be decided before operation to give the patient moderate or deep sedation. Benzodiazepines are the most popular drugs for this purpose. They should be given in small IV increments, e.g. diazepam 1 mg every 30 s, until the desired level of sedation is reached. Intravenous chlormethiazole (0.8% as an infusion) is also very useful as the depth of sedation can be easily and quickly modified by adjustment of the infusion rate. Unlike when benzodiazepines are used, recovery to full lucidity will occur within minutes of stopping the infusion.

8. The patient's blood pressure should be carefully monitored, particularly with spinal or epidural block. Conscious patients tolerate decreases in their arterial pressure badly. Even a modest degree of hypotension may trigger a vasovagal attack with bradycardia (or even transient cardiac arrest), extreme hypotension, unconsciousness, nausea and vomiting.

9. Postoperatively patients with epidural or spinal blocks should be under medical and nursing observation until the local anaesthesia has worn off.

Concomitant general anaesthesia

General anaesthesia used alone has to meet a triad of requirements, namely, unconsciousness, analgesia and relaxation. The last two are usually achieved with specific drugs, i.e. opioids and muscle relaxants. As regional anaesthesia can provide analgesia (which is much superior in quality to that of opioids) and relaxation (confined to the operative area and not involving the muscles of respiration), the addition of a light general anaesthetic to a regional technique is quite logical. The following advantages accrue:

1. A patient's preference to be unconscious can be met. If the local anaesthesia is not adequate for any reason, the patient will be unaware of it though it will be obvious to the anaesthetist, who can deal with it appropriately.

2. Deep anaesthesia is not required and recovery of consciousness is rapid. On the other hand most of the agents used for sedation of a conscious patient are only slowly metabolised and complete recovery may be delayed for many hours.

3. Time is saved because preparations for the operation, e.g. positioning, cleaning the skin and catheterisation, can be made **before** the local anaesthetic is fully effective.

4. Spontaneous respiration is maintained and there is no requirement for paralysis and artificial ventilation.

5. Most patients will awaken in a pain-free state.

6. The stress on the operating team of having a conscious patient is removed.

7. Sudden hypotension as seen with vasovagal attacks does not occur in anaesthetised patients.

8. Hypotension is well tolerated and can indeed be used where indicated to reduce operative bleeding.

The general anaesthesia should be of the simplest type, with an IV agent for induction, followed by a weak concentration of an inhalational agent. Endotracheal intubation is seldom required provided the airway is kept quite clear. If preferred, a total intravenous anaesthetic can be given.

Monitoring during local/regional anaesthesia

Like all patients being anaesthetised, those receiving local anaesthetics should be under continuous observation. The following are considered the minimal requirements:

Pulse

A palpable pulse gives information on the pulse rate and the presence of arrhythmias and is an indication of arterial pressure and cardiac output, particularly if these change rapidly.

ECG

This accurately calculates heart rate, defines an arrhythmia and may show evidence of myocardial ischaemia. A tachycardia seen during or soon after the injection of local anaesthetic may be due to accidental IV injection if epinephrine has been added to the solution. A slow heart rate (55-65 beats/min) may occur when a high sympathetic block occurs and cardiac accelerator nerves are affected. Marked bradycardia (less than 55 beats/min) should warn of a vaso-vagal attack, if the patient is conscious.

Arterial pressure

Non-invasive monitoring of blood pressure is quite adequate in most cases. An automatic machine has many advantages, particularly if the anaesthetist is working alone.

Respiration

Paralysis of the respiratory muscles, particularly the intercostals, may occur with high spinal or epidural block. This will be suggested by dyspnoea and indrawing of the intercostal muscles during inspiration. If a general anaesthetic is being given then the airway and the volume of gas being shifted during respiration should be checked continuously. Irregularity of breathing and breath holding may indicate inadequacy of analgesia and/or too light anaesthesia.

Blood loss

Patients with widespread sympathetic block are less tolerant of blood loss and appropriate fluid replacement must be timely.

More elaborate invasive monitoring including arterial, central venous, pulmonary artery and wedge pressure, may be required in special circumstances.

Local anaesthetic drugs

All local anaesthetic drugs have a common molecular structure and a similar mode of action. There are many drugs available and they differ to a greater or lesser extent in regard to:

1. Potency
2. Onset time or latency
3. Duration of effect
4. Toxicity

Thus the choice of drug will be mainly influenced by the individual patient's requirements.

Unlike most other drugs, local anaesthetics are applied or injected at their site of action, i.e. close to the nerves to be blocked. As a result their **local** concentration is several orders of magnitude greater than their **plasma** concentration after absorption. This accounts not only for their relative safety if they are properly injected in the correct dose, but also for their potential danger if they are injected IV by accident, or an overdose is given.

Chemical structure

All commonly used local anaesthetics have a three-part structure:
Aromatic ring - Intermediate chain - Amino group.
As the intermediate chain contains either an ester or an amide linkage, they may conveniently be divided into esters and amides.

Ester linkage   - COO -

An ester linkage is relatively unstable and ester local anaesthetics are broken down by hydrolysis both in solution and, following injection, in the plasma by pseudocholinesterase. Thus solutions have a relatively short shelf-life and are difficult to sterilise as heat cannot be used. Because they are broken down in the plasma, they can be relatively non-toxic if this process is rapid, as with procaine and chloroprocaine, but in such cases their duration of effect is also brief.

Amide linkage   - NHCO -

An amide linkage is much more stable than an ester, and the drugs in solution withstand heat sterilisation and changes in pH (which may be necessary when adding epinephrine). Likewise they are not broken down in plasma and must be metabolised by the liver, as little or no drug is excreted unchanged.

Physicochemical properties

Local anaesthetics vary in regard to their lipid/water solubility ratio, their pKa and the degree to which they bind to protein (Table 16:1).

Lipid solubility is the main determinant of potency: the higher the lipid/water partition coefficient, the more potent the drug is likely to be.

Protein binding determines the duration of effect, presumably because highly bound drugs stay in the lipoprotein of nerve membranes longer.

The pKa of a compound determines how much is ionised and how much is unionised when injected into the body. Thus the higher the pKa, the less of the unionised base form is present. As only unionised drug can penetrate nerve membranes, the pKa will affect the speed of onset of the drugs: the lower the pKa, the faster the onset (Table 16:2).

Table 16:2
Relationship of pKa to percent base form and time for 50 percent conduction block in isolated nerve

Agent	pKa	% Base at pH 7.4	Onset (min)
Prilocaine	7.7	35	2-4
Lidocaine	7.7	35	2-4
Etidocaine	7.7	35	2-4
Bupivacaine	8.1	20	5-8
Tetracaine	8.6	5	10-15
Procaine	8.9	2	14-18

Table 16:1
Physicochemical properties of local anaesthetics

Agent	Aromatic Lipophillic	Intermediate Chain	Amine Hydro-phillic	Molecular Weight (base)	pKa (25°C)	Partition Coeffi-cient	% Protein Binding
Esters							
Procaine	$H-N(H)$—ring—	$COOCH_2CH_2$	$-N(C_2H_5)(C_2H_5)$	236	8.9	0.02	5.8
Tetracaine	$H_9C_4N(H)$—ring—	$COOCH_2CH_2$	$-N(CH_3)(CH_3)$	264	8.6	4.1	75.6
Chloroprocaine	$H-N(H)$—ring(Cl)—	$COOCH_2CH_2$	$-N(C_2H_5)(C_2H_5)$	271	8.7	0.14	—
Amides							
Prilocaine	ring CH_3	$NHCOCH(CH_3)$	$-N(H)(C_3H_7)$	220	7.7	0.9	55 approx.
Lidocaine		$NHCOCH_2$	$-N(C_2H_5)(C_2H_5)$	234	7.7	2.9	64.3
Mepivacaine	ring $(CH_3)(CH_3)$	$NHCO$	N-ring CH_3	246	7.6	0.8	77.5
Bupivacaine		$NHCO$	N-ring C_4H_9	288	8.1	27.5	95.6
Etidocaine		$NHCOCH(C_2H_5)$	$-N(C_2H_5)(C_3H_7)$	276	7.7	141	94

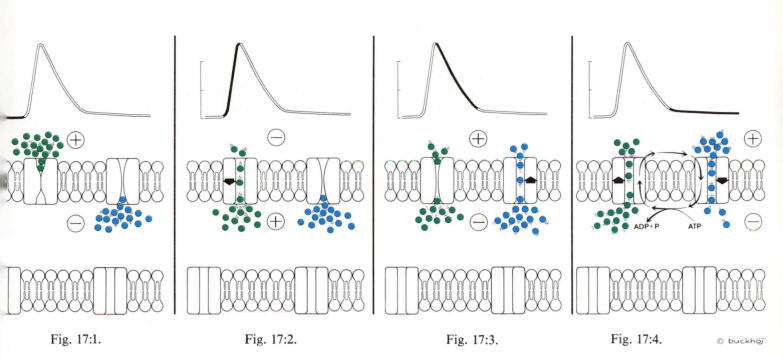

Fig. 17:1. Fig. 17:2. Fig. 17:3. Fig. 17:4. © buckhöj

Mode of action

Local anaesthetics cause a reversible block to the conduction of impulses along nerve fibres. A propagated nerve impulse involves a wave of depolarisation, followed by repolarisation, passing along the nerve fibre. In the resting mode, nerve fibres are polarised, with higher concentrations of sodium ions outside than inside the cell, and the reverse for potassium ions (Fig. 17:1).

Depolarisation is caused by a flow of sodium ions through sodium channels in the nerve membrane, from the outside to the inside of the nerve fibres (Fig. 17:2).

Repolarisation involves the flow, in the reverse direction, of potassium ions (Fig. 17:3).

The resultant slight imbalance of ions (too much Na inside and too much K outside) is corrected after repolarisation by ionic pumps (Fig. 17:4).

The electrical spike caused by depolarisation triggers the adjacent membrane, such that the sodium channels in that section of the fibre open in their turn, allowing the inward flow of sodium ions and depolarisation. Thus each depolarisation/repolarisation that occurs triggers a similar process in the adjacent membrane and this passes along the nerve from one end to the other.

Local anaesthetics cause changes in the nerve membrane which prevent depolarisation and thus block nerve propagation, a process termed "stabilising the membrane". They achieve this by preventing the sodium channels opening, thus maintaining the fully polarised state (Fig. 17:5).

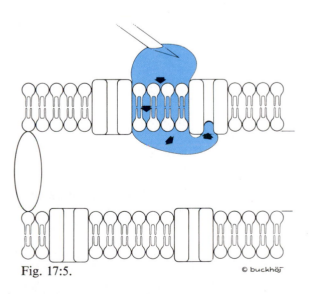

Fig. 17:5. © buckhöj

17

Most local anaesthetics are relatively insoluble in water and are prepared as the soluble hydrochloride salt. When this is injected, it ionises into positively charged anions of the local anaesthetic and negatively charged chloride ions, i.e.

$$LA\ HCl \longrightarrow LAH^+ + Cl^-$$

As the anionic form must also dissociate at the body pH, the following reaction occurs:

$$\underset{\text{Anion}}{LAH^+} \rightleftharpoons \underset{\text{Base}}{LA} + H^+$$

Thus after injection of the hydrochloride salt, both the charged anionic form and the uncharged basic form of the compound rapidly appear. The proportion of charged/uncharged forms depends upon the pKa of the drug. Local anaesthetics have pKa's above 7.4 and the greater the pKa, the greater the amount of the uncharged form that is present.

Only the lipid soluble uncharged form of the drug can penetrate the epineurium and the nerve membrane. The membrane is made up of a lipid bilayer and protein molecules that contain the sodium channels (Fig. 18:1). The axoplasm, however, is a watery milieu and on reaching it after passage through the membrane, the uncharged base must again dissociate and form a mixture of both the charged and uncharged forms. The charged anionic form of the local anaesthetic then gains access to the sodium channels (Fig. 18:2), and renders them incapable of allowing sodium ions to pass through the membrane. Nerve impulses cannot then be propagated. As the block develops depolarisation is, at first slowed and then finally prevented.

Other modes of action

Benzocaine (sodium para-aminobenzoate) does not ionise at body pH and thus only exists in the base form. It can enter the membrane but will not reach the axoplasm. It is thought to act by membrane expansion which will physically occlude the sodium channels, a mechanism similar to that of general anaesthetics on the brain.

Conversely, the biotoxins e.g. tetradotoxin and saxitoxin, which are highly potent local anaesthetics, only exist in the charged ionised form and cannot enter the membrane. To block nerve conduction they must attach themselves to the outer part of the sodium channels. This process is shown in Fig. 18:2.

Fig. 18:1.

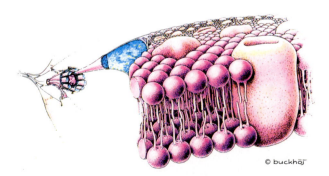

Fig. 18:2.

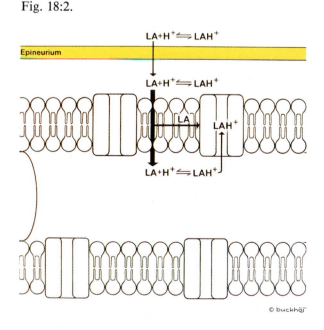

Choice of local anaesthetic drug

In choosing a local anaesthetic drug and the appropriate concentration, the factors to be borne in mind are:

Specific nerves to be blocked

Small nerves are in general much easier to block than large ones. Thus nerve endings and small cutaneous nerves are easily and quickly blocked by low concentrations of drugs given by infiltration. Large nerves with thick perineurium are much more difficult and require high concentrations of drug. However, the large spinal nerves within the subarachnoid space have no perineurium and are easily blocked.

It is generally held that motor fibres are the most difficult to block, followed by somatic sensory and autonomic fibres in descending order. However, there is evidence that the small C fibres, can be relatively resistant to local anaesthetics.

Onset time or latency

A rapid onset may be required, e.g. for an urgent operation or to relieve acute pain. In such cases an agent with a rapid onset can be used or an alternative procedure may be performed, e.g. a spinal block instead of an epidural block.

Epinephrine can decrease latency (vide infra).

Required duration of effect

The duration of local anaesthetics may vary from 30 min to 180 min or longer. Moreover duration is related to the dosage, increasing which gives a longer duration. Clearly the duration should outlast the operation. Thereafter the optimal duration will depend upon the desirability of postoperative analgesia and the need to regain full function.

The duration can be increased by adding epinephrine to the local anaesthetic (vide infra). When very prolonged anaesthesia is required, an indwelling plastic catheter may be used, and repeat injections of local anaesthetic made as required.

For permanent nerve blockade, neurolytic agents such as phenol or alcohol are employed.

Drug properties

Lidocaine HCl

(Carbonated salt also available in some countries).
Short onset, medium duration drug. 0.5-2% for injection, 4-10% for topical application. Used for all forms of regional anaesthesia. Also used for treatment of ventricular arrhythmias.

Prilocaine HCl

Short onset, medium duration drug. Significantly less toxic than lidocaine. Causes methaemoglobinaemia in doses over 600 mg; thus not suitable for continuous analgesia. 0.5-2% for injection. Specially indicated for high dose techniques (e.g. plexus blockade) and for IV regional anaesthesia (Bier's block).

Mepivacaine HCl

Short onset, medium duration drug. Less toxic than lidocaine. 0.5-2% for injection.

Bupivacaine HCl

(Carbonated salt also available in some countries).
Long onset, long duration. 0.125-0.75% for injection (0.75% has short onset). Causes less motor block than most other local anaesthetics at concentrations of 0.5% or less; hence valuable for prolonged analgesia. More cardiotoxic than equipotent concentrations of lidocaine.

Chloroprocaine HCl

Short onset, short acting drug. Low toxicity due to rapid hydrolysis in plasma. 1-3% for injection. Neuropathy has been described, but this was probably due to added metabisulphite and the formulation has now been changed. 3% gives rapid onset for Caesarean sections done with epidural block.

Procaine HCl

Slow onset, short duration drug. Now seldom used. 1-2% for injection. Useful for short duration spinal anaesthesia.

Tetracaine HCl

Slow onset, long duration drug. Main use is in spinal anaesthesia and for topical application. Rather toxic if used for nerve blocks.

Dosage of local anaesthetic drugs

There are few areas in anaesthesia where dosage recommendations are more confused than in regional anaesthesia. This is in large part due to the insistence of the various national pharmacopeias and regulatory authorities on laying down a "maximum recommended dose" for local anaesthetic drugs. Such a restriction does not apply to other classes of drug. The avoidance of toxicity is of course very important, but toxicity seldom arises if the local anaesthetic is injected correctly. The commonest cause of toxicity is accidental IV injection and the "maximum recommended dose" of any local anaesthetic given as a fast bolus injection will still cause overt toxicity with convulsions.

The problem is compounded by the fact that the peak plasma concentration following absorption from a correctly placed injection depends primarily on the site of injection. Thus an intercostal block gives over 3 times the peak concentration that follows a subcutaneous injection in an abdominal field block. Clearly then the "maximum recommended dose" should be adjusted for each site of injection.

Their is a particular difficulty with lidocaine, the most widely used local anaesthetic. Since its introduction over 30 years ago it has been stated that the maximum recommended dose is 200 mg of plain solution and 500 mg of an epinephrine-containing solution. Nothing could be more illogical, the former dose being far too small and the latter making the incorrect assumption that epinephrine allows a 150% increase in dosage. For these reasons the author has doubled the recommended dose for plain solutions of lidocaine, but it should be understood that this is a personal view, not accepted at the present time by the regulatory authorities. Many, and probably most, experts in the field, however, would agree that 400 mg of plain lidocaine will not cause overt toxicity unless it is given accidentally into a blood vessel.

The relative potencies of the common local anaesthetic drugs are given in Table 20:1.

Table 20:1.
Comparative potencies of local anaesthestics (%)

Lidocaine	0.5	1	1.5	2	
Mepivacaine	0.5	1	1.5	2	
Prilocaine	0.5	1	1.5	2	
Bupivacaine	0.125	0.25	0.375	0.5	0.75
Etidocaine	0.25	0.5	0.75	1	1.5
Chloroprocaine	0.5	1	1.5	2	3
Procaine	1	2			

The doses recommended for epidural block (which requires the highest concentration of local anaesthetics), and the doses likely to cause convulsions if given IV by fast bolus injection in adults, are given in Table 21:1. The onset times and durations are also included.

Table 21:1.
Epidural blockade in adults

Drug	Maximum dose epidurally	Toxic dose if IV	Onset to surgical analgesia (min)	Duration (min)
Lidocaine 2%	20 ml (400 mg)	12.5 ml (250 mg)	10-20	90-120
Lidocaine 2% with epinephrine	25 ml (500 mg)	12.5 ml (250 mg)	7-15	120-180
Prilocaine 2%	25 ml (500 mg)	17.5 ml (350 mg)	10-20	90-120
Prilocaine 2% with epinephrine	30 ml (600 mg)	17.5 ml (350 mg)	7-15	120-180
Mepivacaine 2%	25 ml (400 mg)	17.5 ml (350 mg)	10-20	90-120
Mepivacaine 2% with epinephrine	30 ml (600 mg)	17.5 ml (350 mg)	7-15	120-180
Bupivacaine 0.5%	20 ml (100 mg)	16.0 ml (80 mg)	20-40	180-240
Bupivacaine 0.5% with epinephrine	25 ml (125 mg)	16.0 ml (80 mg)	15-30	200-300
Bupivacaine 0.75%	20 ml (150 mg)	11.0 ml (80 mg)	15-30	250-400
Bupivacaine 0.75% with epinephrine	25 ml (182.5 mg)	11.0 ml (80 mg)	10-20	250-450
Etidocaine 1.5%	20 ml (300 mg)	12.0 ml (180 mg)	10-20	200-300
Etidocaine 1.5% with epinephrine	25 ml (375 mg)	12.0 ml (180 mg)	7-15	250-420
Chloroprocaine 3%	20 ml (600 mg)	15.0 ml (450 mg)	10-20	45-60
Chloroprocaine 3% with epinephrine	25 ml (750 mg)	15.0 ml (450 mg)	7-15	60-80

Toxicity of local anaesthetic drugs

There is not a great difference in toxicity between equipotent doses of most local anaesthetics but it is best to use one of low toxicity when large doses are required (e.g. for brachial plexus block) or when IV regional anaesthesia is used.

Systemic toxicity of local anaesthetic drugs

The effect of local anaesthetic drugs on sodium channels in nerve membrane ensures that if toxic effects do occur they will be in organs with excitable membranes, particularly the brain and the myocardium. All those who use potentially toxic doses of local anaesthetics should be aware of the possibility of toxic reactions and know how to recognise and treat them.

The systemic toxicity of local anaesthetic drugs depends upon:

1. Dose

2. Site of injection
   Vascular sites lead to rapid absorption. Thus intercostal injection gives much higher plasma concentrations than subcutaneous injection. Accidental IV injection is the commonest cause of toxicity.

3. Drug used
   The drugs of lowest toxicity are prilocaine, mepivacaine, chloroprocaine and procaine.

4. Speed of injection
   This is only of importance if the drug is given IV, when fast injections will achieve much higher plasma concentrations than slow injections. Injecting small aliquots over several minutes prolongs the administration and will reduce toxicity when high dosage is required, e.g. in epidural, intercostal or major plexus blocks.

5. Addition of epinephrine
   This causes local vasoconstriction and slows absorption. It is more effective at subcutaneous sites than elsewhere but a reduction in the peak concentration of between 20% and 50% may be anticipated with most local anaesthetics.

Signs and symptoms of toxicity

Local anaesthetics have their major toxic effects in the brain and myocardium. The brain is more susceptible than the heart and all the early signs and symptoms are related to CNS toxicity, serious myocardial dysfunction only being seen with excessive plasma concentrations.

Central nervous system toxicity

Central nervous system toxicity involves a spectrum of signs and symptoms from mild to serious. In increasing order of severity, the following may occur:

1. Numbness of the mouth and tongue
2. Lightheadedness
3. Tinnitus
4. Visual disturbance
5. Irrational behaviour and speech
6. Muscle twitching
7. Unconsciousness
8. Generalised convulsions
9. Coma
10. Apnoea

CNS toxicity will be enhanced by acidosis and hypoxia, both of which can occur very rapidly if convulsions appear, when breathing may stop and the excessive muscular activity consumes oxygen stores.

Cardiovascular toxicity

Cardiovascular toxicity is due to slowing of conduction in the myocardium, myocardial depression and peripheral vasodilatation. It is usually only seen clinically after 2-4 times the convulsant dose has been injected. Hypotension, bradycardia and eventually cardiac standstill may occur. An exception to this is with bupivacaine, which can affect conduction within the myocardium at relatively low plasma concentrations. As a result sudden ventricular fibrillation has been seen with this drug after rapid IV injection.

Prevention of toxicity

Local anaesthetic toxicity can be avoided in most cases by a few simple rules:

1. Always use the recommended dose.

2. Aspirate through the needle or catheter before injecting the local anaesthetic.

3. Use a test dose containing epinephrine when appropriate. If the needle or catheter is within a vein, the test dose will produce an acute increase in heart rate 30-45 s after the injection. The duration of the tachycardia is brief and a continuous ECG is recommended.

4. If a large quantity of drug is required or if the drug is given IV on purpose (e.g. for IV regional anaesthesia) use a drug of low toxicity, and divide the dose into smaller aliquots, spreading the time taken for the total injection.

5. Always inject slowly (not faster than 10 ml/min) and maintain verbal contact with the patient, who can report minor symptoms before the entire intended dose is given. Beware of the patient who starts to speak and act irrationally. It is probably due to CNS toxicity but may be mistaken for hysteria.

Treatment of toxicity
Provided the diagnosis is borne in mind, toxicity may be recognised early and effective treatment given without delay. All necessary equipment and drugs should be available **before** injecting local anaesthetic. The two cardinal rules are:

1. Give oxygen, if necessary by artificial respiration using a bag and mask.

2. Stop the convulsions if they continue for more than 15-20 s. To do this an anticonvulsant must be given IV, e.g. thiopental 100-150 mg or diazepam 5-20 mg. The former is usually more readily available and is quicker acting. Some authorities prefer to give succinylcholine 50-100 mg, which will quickly stop the convulsions but will require intubation and artificial ventilation until the effects have worn off.

Toxicity can disappear as quickly as it appears and a decision must then be made whether to postpone surgery, repeat the nerve block, use a different technique (e.g. give a spinal instead of an epidural block) or change to general anaesthesia.

If hypotension and signs of myocardial depression occur, a vasopressor with both α and β-adrenergic activity should be given, e.g. ephedrine 15-30 mg IV. Cardiac standstill must be treated by energetic cardiopulmonary resuscitation including IV or intracardiac epinephrine 1 mg and atropine 0.6 mg. Ventricular fibrillation should be treated by high energy DC conversion plus bretylium 80 mg as an anti-arrhythmic.

Sensitivity to local anaesthetic drugs
Sensitivity or allergy is excessively rare in the case of amide local anaesthetics but is occasionally seen with esters. Other constituents within an ampoule or vial of local anaesthetic e.g. methylparaben, may be responsible for some reactions.

Patients may claim to be sensitive, usually as a result of an unpleasant experience in the course of dental treatment. Most likely the patient fainted or felt faint and this was wrongly labelled as sensitivity.

If there is any doubt the patient should be given a skin test which, if negative, may be followed by a challenge using a small subcutaneous dose. This should only be done in a properly equipped area so that if allergy occurs it can be promptly treated.

Other drugs used in regional anaesthesia

Epinephrine
This may be added to local anaesthetic solutions to increase their effectiveness and to reduce toxicity. It causes a local vasoconstriction and delays absorption from the site of injection. Thus the local anaesthetic is in contact with the target nerves for a longer time. As a result the latency is reduced, the block is more effective and the duration is increased. Slowing the absorption also decreases the peak plasma concentration.

Epinephrine works better at some locations than others, being most effective at subcutaneous sites.

The optimal concentration is 1:200.000, i.e. 5 μg/ml. Local anaesthetics containing epinephrine are available commercially. Alternatively the epinephrine may be added immediately before use, 0.1 ml of 1:1.000 (i.e. 100 μg) being added to 20 ml of local anaesthetic.

It is unwise to inject epinephrine near terminal arteries, e.g. digital arteries, for fear of causing tissue necrosis and gangrene.

Other local vasoconstrictors
Although many agents have been tried, none appears to have any advantage over epinephrine. The only drug which has achieved popularity is felypressin (Octapressin), which is added to prilocaine for dental use.

Parenteral vasopressors

These drugs are used to prevent or correct hypotension resulting from sympathetic blockade in spinal or epidural anaesthesia.

The commonest of these are:

Ephedrine

This is sympathomimetic with both α- and β-receptor activity. Given IV in a dose of 10-15 mg it rapidly (60-90 s) raises arterial pressure, and this effect lasts for 15-30 min. Occasionally larger doses may be required. Given IM it takes 10-15 min to work and it lasts up to 1 h. It is logical, therefore, for a rapid effect and long duration, to give enough drug IV to restore the pressure, and the same dose IM. The IM route can also be used prophylactically to prevent decreases in arterial pressure, e.g. just after injecting the local anaesthetic for spinal or epidural anaesthesia.

Phenylephrine

Phenylephrine is a pure α-receptor agonist, and must be given by IV infusion. 10-20 mg is diluted in 500 ml of saline or dextrose and infused, the dose being titrated to the desired effect.

Methoxamine

Methoxamine (Vasoxine) is an α-receptor agonist and a β-blocker. It raises pressure but slows the heart rate with a consequent decrease in cardiac output. This unusual combination of effects makes it theoretically the best drug to use in patients with coronary insufficiency because it should increase coronary flow (by increasing afterload) and decrease myocardial work (by decreasing cardiac output). Both the IM and IV routes can be used and the dosage is 10-30 mg.

Dihydroergotamine

Dihydroergotamine has been used both to treat and to prevent hypotension. It differs from sympathomimetics in that its main effect is one of vasoconstriction on the venous side of the circulation, causing a decrease in venous capacitance and an increase in venous return. It also causes a mild degree of arteriolar vasoconstriction. Arterial pressure returns towards normal without overshoot or tachycardia. The dose is 0.5-1 mg and it can be used IV or IM. It has been found to decrease liver blood flow.

Complications of regional anaesthesia

The complications of regional anaesthesia may be divided into immediate, intermediate and late.

Immediate complications

Toxic reactions (see p. 22)

(see p. 22)

Hypotension

Hypotension is usually associated with widespread sympathetic blockade and therefore with spinal or epidural block. However, even high blocks involving most of the sympathetic outflow are not associated with severe hypotension in the majority of patients, only about 25% suffering a decrease in systolic pressure greater than 30 mmHg. Additional factors precipitating severe hypotension are:
1. Hypovolaemia
2. Fainting due to vaso-vagal attack
3. Inferior vena caval occlusion in late pregnancy or in the presence of large abdominal tumour.

Hypotension may be prevented by giving a fluid load (e.g., 1 litre of Hartmann's solution) just before performing the block, or by giving a vasopressor. Caval occlusion may be avoided by turning the patient into a semilateral position, or using uterine displacement.

As hypotension only occurs in a minority of patients, some authorities prefer to await its development, and treat it as required, using an IV vasopressor (see p. 24).

(see p. 24)

Respiratory paralysis

Respiratory paralysis can occur with the inadvertent injection of a large quantity of local anaesthetic into the subarachnoid or subdural space instead of the epidural space. Very occasionally it can occur with an unduly high epidural or spinal block. The patient will complain of dyspnoea and the intercostal muscles will be indrawn during inspiration. If the phrenic nerve is paralysed (C3, 4, 5), respiration will cease. Treatment is by artificial respiration until the paralysis wears off.

Patients who faint may also complain of dyspnoea, which is due to air hunger consequent on the very low cardiac output. Extreme bradycardia due to vagal overactivity, in the presence of good respiratory movement, will suggest this diagnosis.

Pain on injection

Acute pain referred to the distribution of the nerve being blocked is a serious event as it indicates an intraneural injection. The injection should be stopped immediately as nerve damage can occur. This shooting type pain should not be confused with the dull aching pain which can occur when large volumes are injected into a confined space, e.g. with brachial plexus block.

Intermediate complications

Motor paralysis

If it occurs within the operative area, muscle paralysis is usually beneficial. However, in the case of epidural and spinal anaesthesia, paralysis of the lower limbs may be a problem as some patients are disturbed by it, especially if the regional block is being used for prolonged pain relief, e.g. in labour or postoperatively. Reassurance of the patient is essential and the use of lower concentrations of drug at subsequent injections will usually allow more active movement of the lower limbs.

Paralysis of the respiratory muscles is mentioned above.

Urinary retention

The parasympathetic motor nerves to the bladder arise from the spinal segments S2, 3 and 4. The sympathetic sensory nerves enter the spinal cord via T11-L2. Thus spinal and epidural blocks at these levels can cause urinary retention and require bladder catheterisation. As patients may not be aware of their distending bladder, they must be observed both in regard to urinary output and a palpable bladder. Catheterisation is often condemned because of the possibility of urinary infection and bacteraemia. Repeated aseptic catheterisation is thought to carry less risk of infection than continuous drainage, but the great majority of patients will suffer little or no harm from catheterisation. Many pelvic and perineal operations require catheterisation regardless of the anaesthesia. Prophylactic antibiotics will prevent infection becoming established.

Late complications

Neurological damage

Neurological damage which may be long-lasting or even permanent is the most feared complication of regional anaesthesia. There are several causes for such damage occurring. (Table 25:1).

Table 25:1
Summary of various types of neurological damage following epidural blockade

Pathology	Cause	Onset	Clinical Features	Outcome
Spinal nerve neuropathy	Trauma (needle, catheter, injection)	0-2 days	Pain during insertion of needle or catheter. Pain on injection. Paraesthesia, pain and numbness over distribution of spinal nerve.	Recovery 1-12 weeks
Anterior spinal artery sydrome	Arteriosclerosis Hypotension	Immediate	Postoperative painless paraplegia.	Painless paraplegia.
Adhesive arachnoiditis	Irritant injectate	0-7 days	Pain on injection. Variable degree of neurological deficit. Often progressive with with pain and paraplegia.	May progress to severe disability pain and paralysis.
Space-occupying lesion (haematoma or abscess)	Hypocoagulation Bacteraemia	0-2 days	Severe backache postoperatively with progressive paraplegia.	Requires immediate surgery, otherwise paraplegia.

Should a neurological complication occur, or be suspected, an expert neurological opinion should be urgently sought. If a space-occupying lesion is suspected, an emergency laminectomy may be necessary. Otherwise a careful history and examination will elucidate the diagnosis and determine the presence and extent of any pre-existing disease.

The main causes of neurological problems are:

Nerve trauma
Apart from the damage to nerve fibres caused by a needle or catheter entering a nerve, the injection of local anaesthetic directly into a nerve can physically disrupt the fibres and may lead to neuropathy.

Anterior spinal artery syndrome
This causes paraplegia and is due to occlusion or inadequate flow in the artery of Adamkiewicz, which supplies the lower third of the spinal cord. The main cause of inadequate flow is hypotension in the presence of local arteriosclerosis.

Adhesive arachnoiditis
This may follow the injection of an irritant or infected solution into the epidural or subarachnoid space.

Space-occupying lesion
A space-occupying lesion in the spinal canal, e.g. haematoma or abscess, can cause paraplegia, and may or may not be associated with the injection of local anaesthetic.

Pneumothorax
Pneumothorax is a complication of intercostal nerve block and supraclavicular brachial plexus block. It should be kept in mind after performing these blocks. A chest X-ray will quickly make the diagnosis. Treatment will depend upon the amount of air in the pleural cavity and the adequacy of respiratory function.

Headache
Headache can follow the piercing of the dura mater in the course of spinal anaesthesia or when it is punctured accidentally during attempted epidural block. The headache is due to low cerebrospinal fluid pressure. Treatment is given on p. 176.

Drug nomenclature

Throughout this book we have used the World Health Organisation's International Non-proprietary Name (INN) convention. The alternative names of the various drugs, whether proprietary or generic, are given in Table 27:1.

Table 27:1
Drug nomenclature

INN	Other names
Local anaesthetics	
Bupivacaine	Marcaine, Sensorcaine, Carbostesin
Chloroprocaine	2-Chlorprocaine, Nesacaine
Etidocaine	Duranest
Lidocaine	Lignocaine, Xylocaine
Mepivacaine	Carbocaine
Prilocaine	Citanest
Procaine	Novocaine
Tetracaine	Amethocaine, Anethaine, Pontocaine, Pantocaine
Vasopressors & Sympathomimetics	
Epinephrine	Adrenaline
Ephedrine	-
Methoxamine	Vasoxine, Vasoxyl
Norepinephrine	Noradrenaline, Levophed
Phenylephrine	Neosynephrine
Opioids	
Fentanyl	Sublimaze
Hydromorphone	Dilaudid
Methadone	Amidone, Phenodone, Physeptone, Dolophine
Morphine	-
Naloxone	Narcan
Pethidine	Meperidine, Demerol, Dolantin
Other drugs	
Chlormethiazole	Heminevrin, Hemineurin
Diazepam	Valium
Midazolam	Hypnovel
Oxytocin	Syntocinon, Syntometrine, Uteracon
Temazepam	Normison, Euhypros
Thiopental	Pentothal, Thiopentone

Aids to regional anaesthesia

Because it is necessary with many techniques of regional anaesthesia to inject the local anaesthetic solution as close as possible to the appropriate nerves, several methods are available to help the anaesthetist determine the anatomy accurately.

Elicitation of paraesthesia

If a sensory nerve is touched by a hypodermic needle a paraesthesia in the distribution of the nerve will occur. While this is used to identify the nerve for many blocks it is important not to damage the nerve. Thus long bevelled and very sharp needles are to be avoided. Patient cooperation is of course essential.

Nerve stimulator

By passing small electric pulses down the injection needle, the proximity of the needle point to the nerve can be determined, as twitching in the muscles supplied by the nerve begins as the needle approaches it. Provided excess current is not used, this is not painful for the patient. The position in which the twitch is maximal gives the nearest position to the nerve. Nerve stimulation can be used even in heavily sedated patients. The following points must be borne in mind:

1) The nerve stimulator (Fig. 28:1) must be able to deliver impulses of varying intensity from 0.2-5.0 mA at a frequency of 1 per second and a duration of 50- 200 μs. Several machines are available commercially and those used for determining neuromuscular block are usually satisfactory. Approximate location to within 2 cm of the nerve is achieved using a current of 2-5 mA but this should be reduced to 0.2-0.5 mA when approaching closer to the nerve. The current used will depend upon the duration of the stimulating impulse and it should therefore be adjustable and indicated on a dial or digital display.

2) While an ordinary needle can be used, it is better to employ an insulated needle (Fig. 28:2) and it should be connected to the negative electrode. This ensures greater accuracy. The needle may be specially designed for the purpose but an IV needle and plastic cannula can easily be adapted to receive the electrical current. (Remember that IV needles are very sharp.)

3) Once muscle twitching in the nerve distribution at low current is obtained, the injection of 1 ml of local anaesthetic (or any other solution) will immediately abolish the twitch, confirming close proximity between the needle tip and the nerve.

The nerve stimulator can also be used to elicit paraesthesia when the nerve to be blocked does not contain motor fibres, e.g. the ophthalmic and maxillary divisions of the trigeminal nerve. It requires a higher current than that which produces muscular twitching.

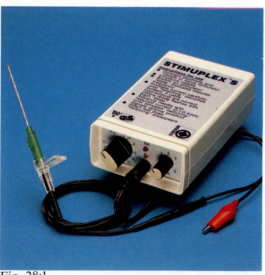

Fig. 28:1.

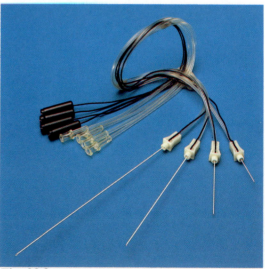

Fig. 28:2.

Ultrasound

Some nerves have a close anatomical relationship to large arteries, identification of which is essential to success. In thin people this seldom presents a problem, but it can be quite difficult in muscular or fat patients. Excessive finger pressure used to feel the arterial pulsations can distort the position of the artery. Ultrasound will identify the correct position of the artery to within 1-2 mm without distortion and is particularly useful in brachial plexus block and femoral nerve block.

Immobile needle

With many nerve blocks it is essential that, having located the nerve, the needle is not moved during the injection. It is therefore not possible to hold the needle, connect the syringe and make the injection oneself. However, using a plastic extension tube to join the needle to the syringe, it is easy for the injection to be made by an assistant without the anaesthetist having to move either hand (Fig. 29:1).

Radiological control

For some blocks where a neurolytic procedure is to be carried out, e.g. coeliac plexus block, it is essential to confirm the accurate placement of the neurolytic agent. This can be greatly simplified by the use of an image intensifier. The position of the needle tip can be checked (Figs. 29:2 and 29:3), and when considered satisfactory, a small amount of radio-opaque dye is injected to eliminate misplacement. The main injection is only made when the correct position has been confirmed. Radio-opaque dye added to the neurolytic agent will also act as a useful check that the injection has been made in the correct location.

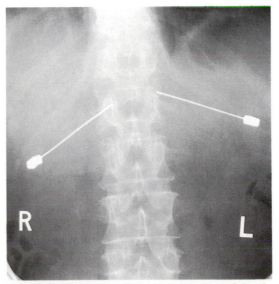

Fig. 29:2. Courtesy of Dr. G.L.M. Carmichael

Fig. 29:3. Courtesy of Dr. G.L.M. Carmichael

Fig. 29:1.

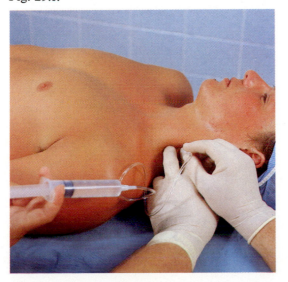

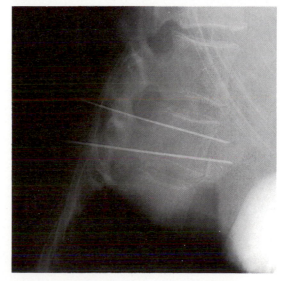

Suggested further reading

Charlton JE (1987). The management of regional anaesthesia. In Principles and Practice of Regional Anaesthesia. Eds Wildsmith JAW and Armitage EN. Churchill Livingstone, Edinburgh.

Covino BG and Vassallo HE (1976). Local anaesthetics: Mechanisms of action and clinical use. Grune and Stratton, New York.

Reiz S and Nath S (1986). Cardiotoxicity of local anaesthetic agents. Br J Anaesth 58, 736.

Scott DB (1986). Toxic effects of local anaesthetic agents on the central nervous system. Br J Anaesth 58, 732.

Tucker GT and Mather LE (1988). Properties, absorption and disposition of local anaesthetic agents. In Neural Blockade, 2nd edition. Eds Cousins MJ and Bridenbaugh PO. Lippincott, Philadelphia. p. 47.

Mucous membranes

Most local anaesthetics cause anaesthesia of mucous membranes when applied topically. They can be used in this way for several diverse procedures, such as urethral catheterisation or corneal analgesia, to render the instrumentation or surgery free from pain.

While it is common to use comparatively high concentrations of local anaesthetic drugs, e.g. lidocaine 4%, this is not always necessary, 0.5% bupivacaine for instance being quite effective for this purpose.

Absorption from mucous membranes is slow and incomplete and most of the local anaesthetic is removed physically from the application site, e.g. by tears if placed in the eye or by swallowing if sprayed into the mouth and throat. As a result the plasma concentrations are much lower than when the drugs are injected. Nevertheless, the amount of drug being administered should be calculated by the anaesthetist.

Topical anaesthesia of the bronchial tree is a special case because rapid and complete absorption can occur if the local anaesthetic reaches the smaller bronchioles and the alveoli, when the rise in plasma concentration will resemble an intravenous injection. However, this is only likely if the patient has been rendered incapable of coughing, e.g. by muscle relaxant drugs. The conscious patient who can still cough will eject the local anaesthetic from the tracheo-bronchial tree and then swallow it. This is in contrast to spraying the paralysed patient prior to endotracheal intubation, when much higher plasma concentrations may be measured.

Swallowing local anaesthetic is relatively safe as the amide drugs will undergo rapid first pass metabolism in the liver after absorption from the gut. However, it is still possible to experience a mild degree of CNS toxicity if the amount swallowed approaches 1 g, presumably due to the breakdown products of metabolism.

The local anaesthetics available for topical anaesthesia of mucous membranes are:

1. Lidocaine 4% solution for use with a spray. Maximum recommended dose 200 mg.
2. Lidocaine 10% as a metered aerosol delivering 10 mg with each activation. Maximum recommended dose 200 mg (20 puffs).
3. Lidocaine 2% gel for urethral analgesia. Maximum dose 10-15 ml (200-300 mg).
4. Cocaine 5-10% is still prefered by some because unlike lidocaine it causes local vasoconstriction.

Intact skin

Skin is very resistant to substances applied topically, though transcutaneous absorption can occur slowly with some substances. To be effective the absorption of local anaesthetics must be sufficient to block the nerve endings found in the epidermis. In general local anaesthetics are ineffective or unreliable for this purpose.

By mixing the pure base of lidocaine with that of prilocaine (both of which are solids at room temperature) an oily liquid is formed, i.e. a eutectic mixture. This can then be emulsified into small droplets which contain much higher (80%) concentrations of local anaesthetic than is possible with hydrochloride solutions (20%). Thus although the concentration of local anaesthetic in the emulsion is only 5%, the concentration in each droplet which comes into contact with the skin is 80%. This eutectic mixture of local anaesthetic (EMLA®) can be applied to intact skin under an occlusive dressing and if left for at least 1 h, will produce anaesthesia of the superficial layers of the skin (Fig. 33:1).

The main indication for EMLA® is to remove the pain of needle puncture (Figs. 33:2 and 3), but it has been used successfully for split skin grafting and mollusc removal (Figs. 33:4 and 5). It should not be used when full thickness skin incisions are to be made.

Absorption is slow and plasma concentrations remain low even after many hours of application. However, the use of large quantities in small children is not advised because the absorption of prilocaine leads to the accumulation of its metabolite orthotoluidine, which can cause methaemoglobinaemia.

Fig. 33:1, Courtesy of Astra.
1. Uptake of local anaesthetic
2. Hydrated straum corneum
3. EMLA Cream
4. Occlusive foil

Figs 33:2-3.
Photo A. Villani, Courtesy of Astra.

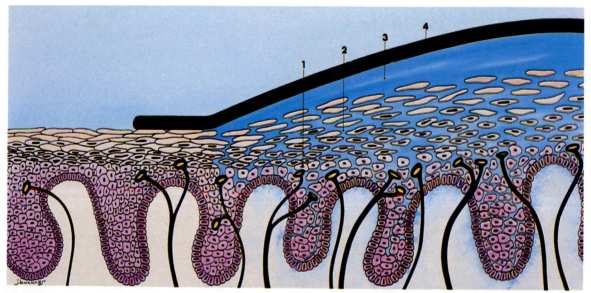

Fig. 33:1.

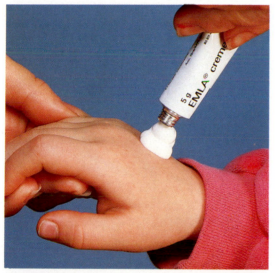

Fig. 33:2.

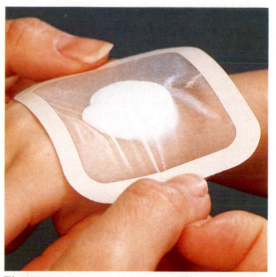

Fig. 33:3.

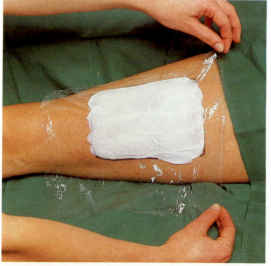

Fig. 33:4.

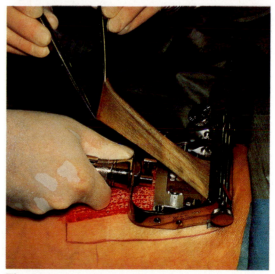

Fig. 33:5.

Anaesthesia for laryngoscopy, bronchoscopy and awake intubation of the trachea

Anaesthesia of the upper airways is relatively simple to achieve with topical anaesthesia.

The mouth may be sprayed under direct vision (Fig. 35:3). The nose may also be sprayed after which it can be packed with a gauze strip soaked in local anaesthetic.

Flexible bronchoscopes are passed down the nose to enter the pharynx (Fig. 35:4). Further doses of local anaesthetic may be sprayed directly at the structures visible through the bronchoscope using the suction port. This of course includes the larynx, through which the instrument must be advanced to reach the trachea, where further local anaesthetic is sprayed to minimise coughing during the procedure.

Reaching the larynx with non-flexible instruments requires the use of a laryngoscope. Indirect laryngoscopy with a mirror is very simple and allows both examination of the larynx and the ability to apply more local anaesthetic.

Direct laryngoscopy is somewhat traumatic and involves an inferior and anterior movement of the tongue to reveal the larynx. Adequate spraying of the pharynx is essential. The larynx, once revealed, is then available for spraying. A fine cannula may be passed through the vocal cords to spray the lower larynx and the trachea (Fig. 35:1).

More direct application of local anaesthetic to the larynx and trachea can be achieved through a needle inserted into the upper trachea, passing through the cricothyroid ligament (Fig. 35:2). The ligament is easily identified and a needle inserted in the midline, perpendicular to the trachea, is advanced until it enters the upper trachea. 2-3 ml of local anaesthetic injected with a syringe will induce coughing which will distribute the drug over the vocal cords and the pharynx. Direct laryngoscopy and passage of an endotracheal tube can then be performed.

The larynx may also be anaesthetised by blocking of the superior laryngeal nerves (see p. 72).

Fig. 35:1. Courtesy of Astra.
1. *Vestibular fold*
2. *Vocal fold*
3. *Superior laryngeal nerve*

Fig. 35:2.
1. *Trachea*
2. *Thyroid cartilage*
3. *Hyoid bone*
4. *Cricoid cartilage*
5. *Cricothyroid ligament*
6. *Thyrohyoid membrane*

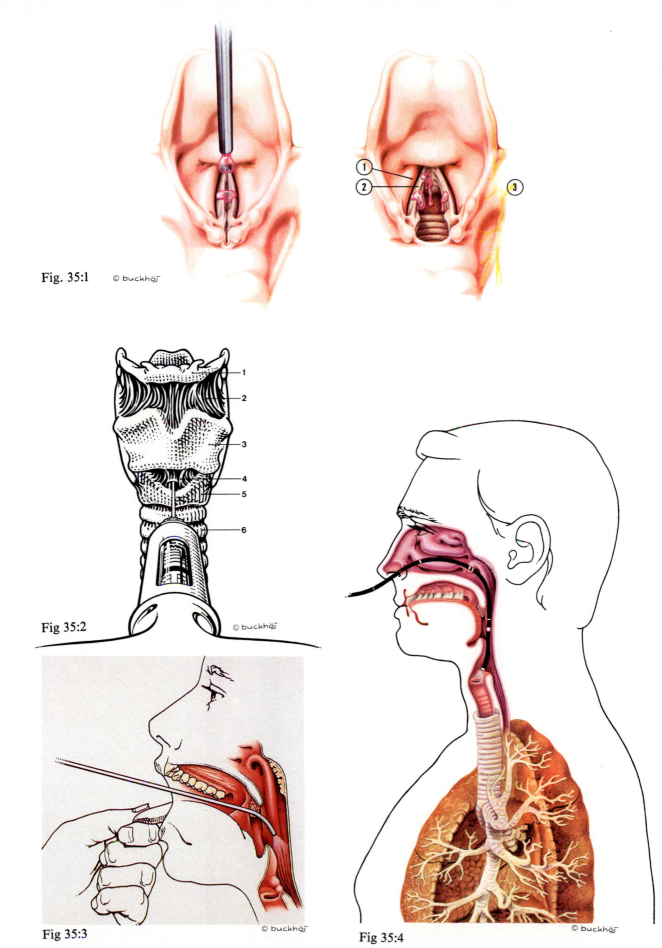

Fig. 35:1   © buckhöj

Fig 35:2   © buckhöj

Fig 35:3   © buckhöj

Fig 35:4   © buckhöj

Nasal anaesthesia

Local anaesthesia of the nasal cavities will reduce considerably the pain and discomfort of nasal operations, many of which can be performed with the patient awake. Even when general anaesthesia is used, the application of local anaesthetic will reduce the pain and therefore the amounts of general anaesthetic required. It will also provide several hours of postoperative analgesia.

Nasal septum

The nasal cavity is well supplied with blood vessels and operations are associated with considerable blood loss, obstructing the surgeon's view. The use of epinephrine with the local anaesthetic will greatly reduce this blood loss. To produce a 1:200.000 concentration of epinephrine, 0.1 ml of 1:1.000 (100 μg) should be added to 20 ml of local anaesthetic.

For operations on the septum, a submucous injection of local anaesthetic containing epinephrine can be made **after** the mucous membrane has been anaesthetised.

Method

1. Spray the nose bilaterally using 4% lidocaine. (Fig. 37:1).

2. Pack the nose with gauze tampons soaked in 4% lidocaine containing 1:200.000 epinephrine. Leave for 10 min (Fig. 37:2).

3. Inject 5 ml of 1% lidocaine containing 1:200.000 epinephrine submucously on each side of the septum immediately before beginning surgery (Fig. 37:3).

Maxillary sinuses

Simple puncture of the sinuses to allow drainage of pus can be performed after direct nasal application of 4% lidocaine with epinephrine 1:200.000, as described above.

Radical operations such as the Caldwell-Luc are performed through the anterior wall of the sinus above the roots of the upper teeth. This area is supplied by the superior dental plexus and is easily anaesthetised with a submucous injection above the canine tooth into the buccal sulcus. Following anaesthesia of the cavity using steps 1 and 2 above, 5 ml of 1% lidocaine is injected as shown in Fig. 37:4.

Fig. 37:1. Courtesy of Astra.
1. Anterior ethmoidal nerve
2. Lateral posterior superior nasal nerves
3. Pterygopalatine ganglion
4. Posterior inferior nasal branches

Fig. 37:4. Courtesy of Astra.

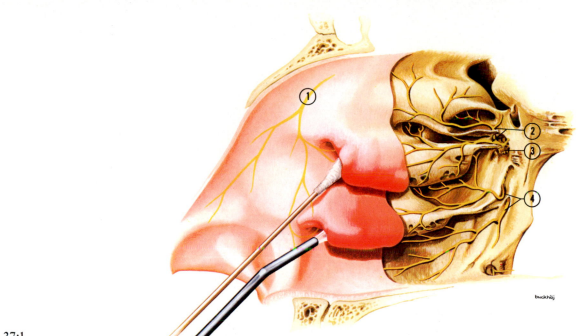

Fig 37:1.

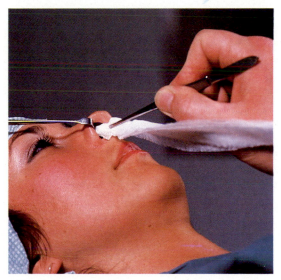

Fig. 37:2.

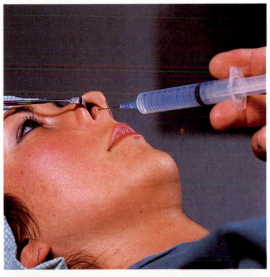

Fig 37:3.

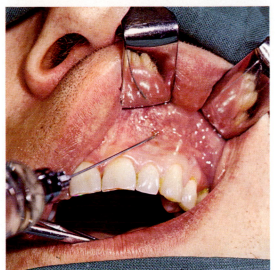

Fig. 37:4.

Urethral anaesthesia

It is a simple matter to anaesthetise the urethra by local application of local anaesthetic. This is usually done with lidocaine gel. It should be remembered that only the lining of the urethra will be anaesthetised, there being no such effect on the bladder sphincter. Passage of an instrument through the sphincter should be gentle and slow to avoid discomfort.

For obvious reasons the female urethra (Fig. 39:1) is easier to anaesthetise than the male (Fig. 39:2), 5 ml of gel being quite sufficient.

To properly anaesthetise the male urethra, the gel must reach along the whole length of the urethra and it must be given sufficient time to achieve its full effect (not less than 5 min). Merely lubricating a catheter or cystoscope with lidocaine gel will have little or no effect. Likewise the passage of an instrument too soon after instillation of the gel will often cause discomfort.

20 ml of 2% lidocaine gel is the recommended dose and this can be put into the urethra with special applicators such as the "accordian" (Fig. 39:3). The gel should be massaged up the urethra to be sure it reaches the membranous and prostatic parts. A penile clamp is then applied and painless instrumentation can occur after 5-10 min. (Fig. 39:4).

Absorption of local anaesthetic from the urethra is minimal though care should be taken if there is active infection.

Fig. 39:3.
Photo A. Villani, Courtesy of Astra.

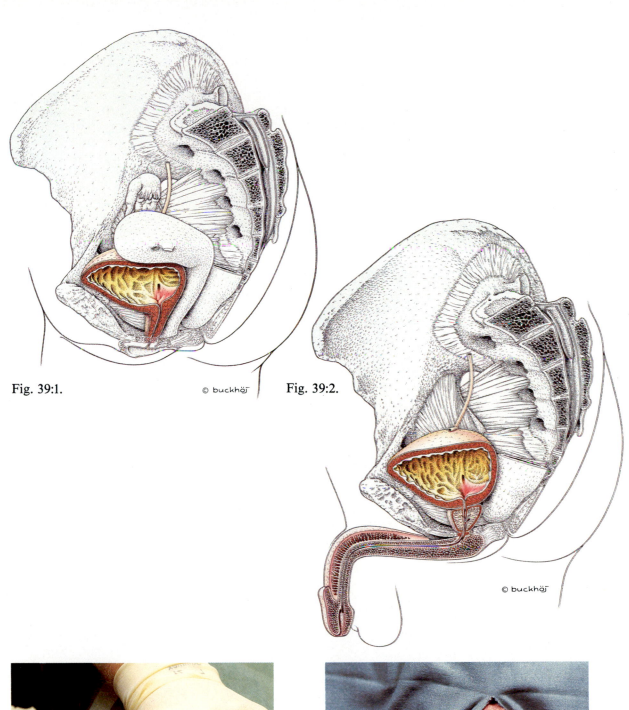

Fig. 39:1.

© buckhöj

Fig. 39:2.

© buckhöj

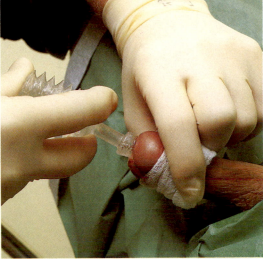

Fig. 39:3.

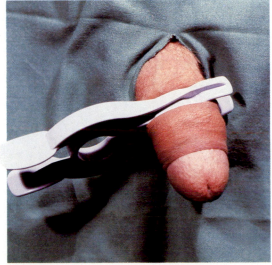

Fig 39:4.

39

Arthroscopy of the knee joint

Although synovial membrane is very sensitive, it is easy to anaesthetise with relatively low concentrations of local anaesthetic applied topically. Thus 0.5% lidocaine or 0.125% bupivacaine installed into the knee joint will allow painless arthroscopy to be carried out.

When done under general anaesthesia it is usual to employ a tourniquet on the thigh to prevent bleeding during arthroscopy or during any surgical manoeuvre, such as removal of a meniscus through the arthroscope. If local anaesthetic is being used in an awake patient, then a tourniquet cannot be used. Nethertheless bleeding can be reduced to a minimum by adding epinephrine to the local anaesthetic solution. Absorption from the synovial membrane is very limited and toxicity either from local anaesthetic or the epinephrine are not to be feared.

If the surgery is to be carried out through the arthroscope, it is necessary to be able to flush the joint with fluid to wash out blood or tissue debris which can obscure the view. Fortunately flushing does not appear to have any marked effect on the anaesthesia, though some prefer to add local anaesthetic to the irrigation fluid. If anaesthesia becomes insufficient during the procedure, it is easy to stop the irrigation temporarily and to inject a new dose of local anaesthetic into the joint to re-anaesthetise it.

Local instillation of local anaesthetic can also be used as an adjuct to general anaesthesia and will reduce the amount of general anaesthetic required.

Patient position
Supine with the knees flexed at right angles.

Landmarks
The patella bone and tendon.

Neddle insertion
The most reliable method of entering the joint is to go behind the patella. A wheal is raised 1 cm above the upper border of the patella and a needle inserted downwards until it is 1 cm below the upper border. (Fig. 41:1).

A subcutaneous infiltration will also be required along the line of insertion of the arthroscope, which is usually lateral to the patella tendon. (Fig. 41:2).

Drugs and dose
50-60 ml of 0.5% lidocaine or 0.125% bupivacaine. Epinephrine may be added to a concentration of 1:200.000 i.e. 0.25 ml of 1 in 1.000 (250 μg) in 50 ml. The joint will be seen to swell with this volume. Flexion and extension of the knee will help the spread of solution to all parts of the joint. 3-5 minutes should be allowed for anaesthesia to develop, after which arthroscopy can proceed (Fig. 41:3 and 41:4).

Complications
If the view through the arthroscope is obscured by blood or debris, the knee may be flushed, either intermittently or continously, with saline.

Sometimes tension or spasm in the quadriceps muscles can interfere with the arthroscopy, and some authorities precede the procedure with a femoral block (see p. 122).

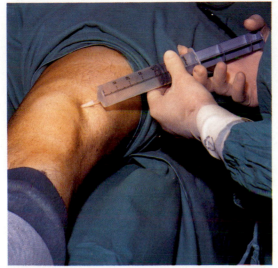

Fig. 41:1.

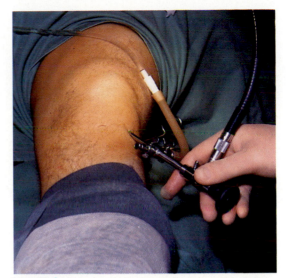

Fig. 41:2.

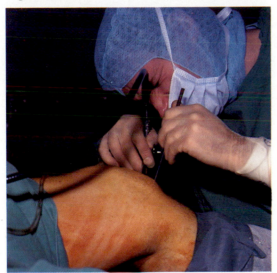

Fig. 41:3.

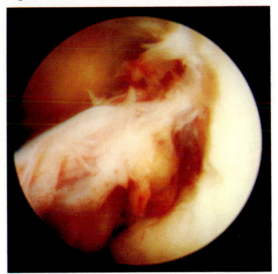

Fig. 41:4.

Topical anaesthesia in ophthalmology

See p. 80.

Local infiltration

Many operations can be performed under direct infiltration of local anaesthetic at the operative site. Dilute solutions are quite effective and although large volumes may be required, toxicity is not a high risk, especially if epinephrine is added.

The simplest way is to inject the local anaesthetic step by step as the operation proceeds. Thus as the structures are exposed, they can be infiltrated under direct vision. For superficial operations such as herniorrhaphy, the whole procedure can usually be carried out after the initial infiltration, but if the patient complains of discomfort during the operation, more anaesthetic can be injected into the sensitive area.

Local infiltration for inguinal and femoral hernia repair

The repair of a hernia is easily accomplished by local infiltration combined with blockade of the ilioinguinal and iliohypogastric nerves. For the surgery to be painless it is necessary for the skin and muscle layers to be infiltrated together with anaesthesia of the hernial sac (which is parietal peritoneum) and, in males, the spermatic cord.

Anatomy
(Fig. 45:1).

Precautions
If possible the hernia should be reduced before starting the anaesthesia to avoid needle puncture of any gut lying within the hernial sac. If the hernia is strangulated, it may prove necessary to resect gut. This can be done with local infiltration, but will need further infiltration of the mesentery of the bowel under direct vision. Provided the patient is not dehydrated as a result of the strangulation, it may be better to consider a spinal anaesthetic.

If the hernia is very large, it may also be much easier to repair with spinal anaesthesia.

Technique for inguinal hernia repair
1a. Raise a skin wheal 2 cm medial to the anterior superior iliac spine. Through this insert a needle towards the umbilicus and infiltrate (5 ml) subcutaneously (Figs. 45:2 and 3).

1b. Repeat this injection (5 ml) deep to the external oblique anastomosis.

1c. Direct the needle in the opposite direction so that it contacts the pelvic bone 1 cm deep to the anterior superior iliac spine. Inject 5 ml of solution, withdrawing the needle slowly. This injection should be made into the muscle tissue of the external and internal oblique muscles and the transversus. It will block the ilioinguinal and iliohypogastric nerves.

2a. Palpate the internal inguinal ring and inject 5 ml of solution into it (Fig. 45:3).

2b. Infiltrate 5-10 ml subcutaneously along the line of the incision (Fig. 45:3).

3. In males, pick up the spermatic cord at the external inguinal ring and inject 5 ml of solution directly into it. Apart from the normal contents of the spermatic cord, it will also contain the hernial sac. In females inject 5 ml above and medial to the pubic tubercle. (Fig. 45:4).

4. Further infiltration may be made under direct vision during the operation.

Technique for femoral hernia repair
Use the same technique as for inguinal hernia repair, omitting step 3.

Drugs and dose
Lidocaine 0.5%, prilocaine 0.5%, mepivacaine 0.5%, bupivacaine 0.125%. Epinephrine 1:200.000 may be added. Total dose not to exceed 60 ml in an adult.

Fig. 45:1.
1. *External oblique muscle*
2. *Internal oblique muscle*
3. *Anterior superior iliac spine*
4. *Transversus abdominis muscle*
5. *Iliohypogastric nerve*
6. *Inguinal ligament*
7. *Ilioinguinal nerve*
8. *Genital branch of the genitofemoral nerve*
9. *Spermatic cord*
10. *Pubic tubercle*
11. *Superficial inguinal ring*
12. *Inguinal hernia*
13. *Saphenous opening*

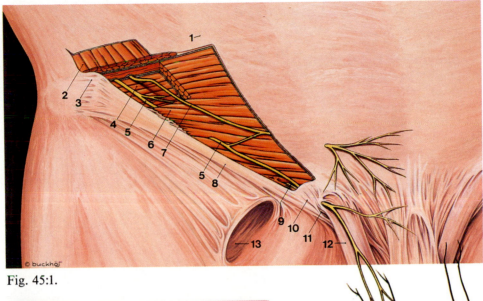

Fig. 45:1.

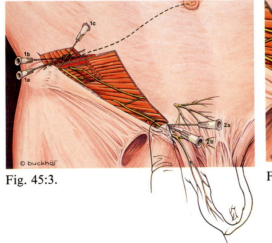

Fig. 45:2.

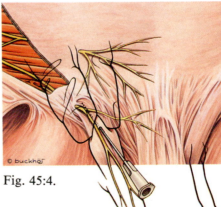

Fig. 45:3.

Fig. 45:4.

45

Local infiltration for Caesarean section

While epidural or spinal blockade are widely used for Caesarean section, as is general anaesthesia, circumstances sometimes arise in which it is hazardous to use any of these methods. e.g. in cases of failed intubation, spinal deformity, massive bleeding or neuromuscular disease. It is worth bearing in mind that the operation can be performed using local infiltration with the mother conscious.

Anatomy
Fig. 47:1.

Method
The best results are obtained by infiltrating local anaesthetic as the operation proceeds. Thus all the injections may be given into the appropriate locations under direct vision. A little time (30-60 s) should be allowed for each injection to become effective.

1. Infiltrate the skin and subcutaneous tissue in the line of the incision (15-20 ml). Incise the skin and expose the rectus sheath (47:2).

2. Infiltrate deep to the rectus sheath on the side of the proposed incision through the sheath (10-15 ml) (Figs. 47:3 and 4). The terminal branches of the intercostal nerves pass through the recti muscles and will be blocked, enhancing anaesthesia of the skin.

Fig. 47:1.
1. *Anterior layer of rectus sheath*
2. *Rectus abdominis muscle*
3. *Posterior layer of rectus sheath*
4. *Linea alba*
5. *Median umbilical ligament*
6. *Parietal peritonium*
7. *Foetus*
8. *Anterior cutaneous branch of the intercostal nerve*
9. *Uterine wall*
10. *Transversalis fascia*

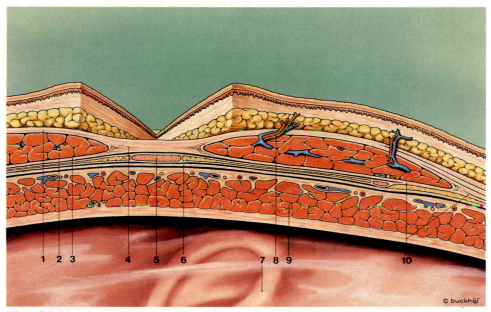

Fig. 47:1.

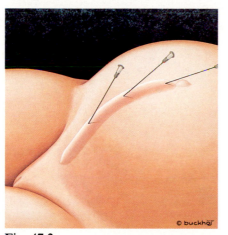

Fig. 47:2.

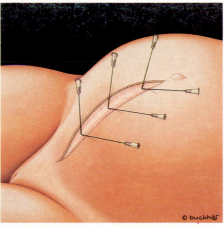

Fig. 47:3.

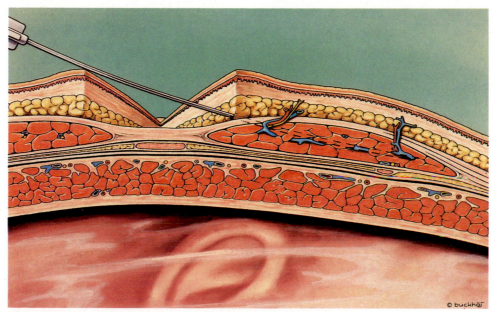

Fig. 47:4.

3. Incise the rectus sheath (Fig. 49:1) and gently retract the rectus muscle to expose the posterior rectus sheath, which ends at the arcuate line midway between the umbilicus and the pubis.

4. Infiltrate below the posterior rectus sheath above the arcuate line and directly into the extraperitoneal tissue (transversalis fascia) below the line (10-15 ml). (Fig. 49:2).

5. Open the peritoneal cavity and expose the uterus.

6. Expose the utero-vesical fold of peritoneum and infiltrate it (10-15 ml) (Fig. 49:3). The peritoneum may now be incised and the lower uterine segment exposed by gently pushing away the bladder (Fig. 49:4).

7. Infiltrate the uterine wall along the proposed incision (10-15 ml).

8. Incise the wall and extract the foetus.

9. Complete the operation.

Drugs and dose
Lidocaine 0.5% 60-100 ml, 0.5% mepivacaine, 0.125% bupivacaine. Epinephrine 1:200.000 may be added.

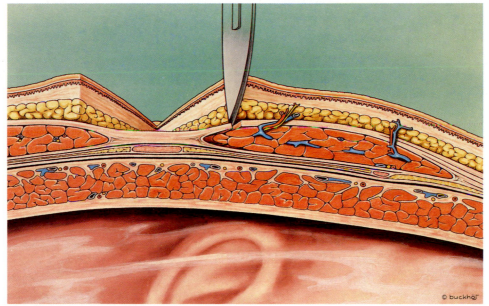

Fig. 49:1.

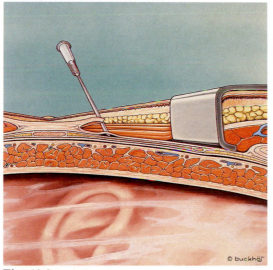

Fig. 49:2.

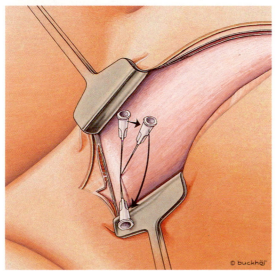

Fig. 49:3.

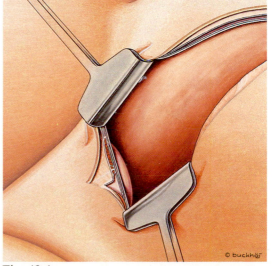

Fig. 49:4.

Intravenous regional anaesthesia (Bier's block)

Intravenous regional anaesthesia is a simple and effective method of producing anaesthesia of the limbs, both upper and lower. It is based on the fact that if the circulation to a limb is occluded and an injection of local anaesthetic is made into a vein distal to that occlusion, the drug will reach the capillaries by retrograde flow and enter the extravascular space. Here it will come into contact with nerve endings and nerve trunks, causing numbness and paralysis of the limb below the tourniquet for the duration of the circulatory occlusion.

Method

Upper limb *primarily*

1. All drugs, oxygen and equipment necessary for the treatment of toxicity should be available. Venous access in the non-operated limb should be established.

2. An inflatable tourniquet is placed around the upper arm over a wool bandage to protect the skin. Ideally, the tourniquet should be one specially designed for the purpose with a gauge and hand pump (Fig. 51:1).

Alternatively, an ordinary sphygmomanometer cuff may be used if essential precautions are taken. It must be very carefully tested for leaks and the connection to the mercury column or pressure gauge must be totally secure. Once the cuff is pressurised, it is vital that deflation below arterial pressure does not occur accidentally. To prevent sudden deflation due to slipping of the cuff, a non-elastic bandage should be wrapped around the cuff (Fig. 51:2).

3. A needle, a 23 gauge butterfly needle (Fig. 51:3) or a small IV plastic cannula, is placed into a vein on the dorsum of the hand and secured to the skin.

4. The limb is exsanguinated of venous blood. This may be done by applying an Esmarch or elastic bandage from the hand up to the blood pressure cuff (Fig. 51:4). In cases of fractures when this process may be painful, the limb may simply be raised vertical for a few minutes to empty the veins as much as possible, without applying the bandage (Fig. 51:5).

5. The blood pressure cuff is then inflated to 250 mmHg or 100 mmHg above systolic pressure, and the Esmarch or elastic bandage below the cuff removed (Fig. 51:6)

6. Local anaesthetic is now injected into the indwelling needle. This injection **should be slow**, not exceeding 1 ml every 2 s. The drug will be seen to enter the capillaries and produce pale areas of skin (Fig. 51:7).

7. At least 10-15 min must be allowed to achieve anaesthesia before beginning the surgical procedure (Fig. 51:8).

8. Following the completion of surgery, and not within 20 min of completing the local anaesthetic injection, the blood pressure cuff may be deflated. The longer the tourniquet is in place, the more local anaesthetic will reach the extracellular space, reducing the amount of drug which will be released on removal of the tourniquet.

9. Normal sensation and muscle function will return within a few minutes, though patchy anaesthesia may remain for up to 60 min.

Drugs and dose

40 ml is usually required in an adult though this should be reduced in children (0.5 ml/kg body weight) or if the limb is clearly small and thin. The solution must be dilute, i.e. 0.5% of prilocaine, lidocaine or mepivacaine. Other agents such as bupivacaine are not recommended nor should epinephrine be added. Remember the drug is being injected intravenously and toxicity can easily occur with accidental deflation of the cuff. Too rapid an injection can produce a high pressure within the veins and drug can escape past the tourniquet. This may also occur if the veins are not emptied before the injection.

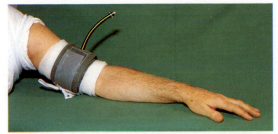

Fig. 51:1.

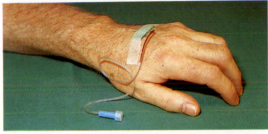

Fig. 51:2.

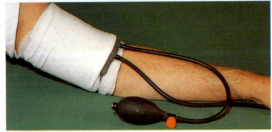

Fig. 51:3.

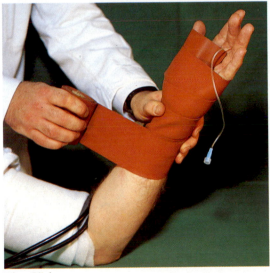

Fig. 51:4.

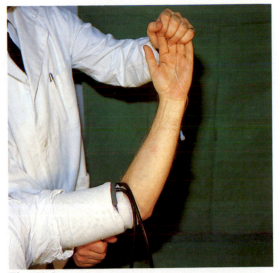

Fig. 51:5.

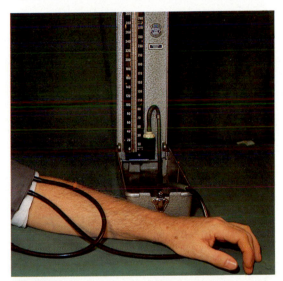

Fig. 51:6.

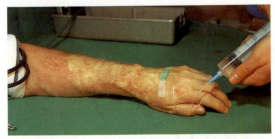

Fig. 51:7.

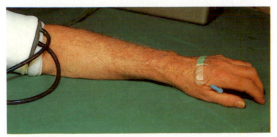

Fig. 51:8.

Lower limb

For lower limb surgery the tourniquet cuff may be placed on the thigh, the calf or the ankle (Fig. 53:1, 2 and 3) depending upon the site of the operation. An intravenous needle or cannula is placed in a vein on the dorsum of the foot. After exsanguinating the limb, the cuff should be inflated to a pressure of 300 mmHg or at least 150 mmHg above the systolic pressure (Fig. 53:1). The procedure is thereafter the same as for the upper limb.

Drugs and dose

With a thigh cuff the dose is 40-60 ml of dilute local anaesthetic 0.5% prilocaine, lidocaine or mepivacaine. With a calf (Fig. 51:2) or ankle (Fig. 51:3) tourniquet the dose is 30 or 20 ml respectively.

Complications

Toxicity

This may be due to accidental deflation of the cuff during or soon after injection of the local anaesthetic. Drug may also pass beneath the inflated tourniquet and reach the systemic circulation during the injection if the limb is not properly exsanguinated before inflating the cuff, and/or the injection is made too rapidly. Both can raise the pressure in the veins to levels above the pressure in the cuff. The signs, symptoms and treatment of toxicity are given on p. 22.

Tourniquet pain

After 20 min or so the inflated tourniquet cuff may become very painful. If a second cuff is placed distal to the original one the tissues beneath it will be anaesthetised. The second cuff may then be inflated painlessly. Once the second cuff has been secured and inflated, the first one may be deflated. Specially designed double cuffs are available.

Suggested further reading:

Duggan J, McKeown DW & Scott DB (1984). Venous pressures in intravanous regional anesthesia. Regional Anesthesia 9. 70.

Holmes C.M. (1988) Intravenous regional neural blockade. In Neural Blockade, 2nd edition Cousins, M.J. & Bridenbaugh, P.O. Lippincott, Philadelphia, p. 443.

Lee A, McKeown DW, Wildsmith JAW (1986). Clinical comparison of equipotent doses of bupivacaine and prilocaine in intravenous regional anesthesia. Regional Anesthesia 11. 102.

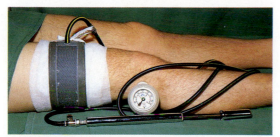

Fig. 53:1.

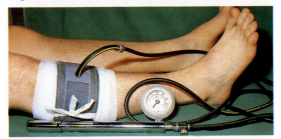

Fig. 53:2.

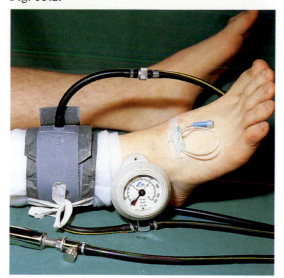

Fig. 53:3.

Peripheral nerve block

Regional anaesthesia of the head and neck

Most operations of the head and neck can be done under regional anaesthesia though in many cases it would not be appropriate, e.g. tonsillectomy in children. However, in the fields of dental, ophthalmological and plastic surgery, there is wide scope for the use of regional techniques, either alone or in combination with sedation or light general anaesthesia. Painful conditions, particularly trigeminal neuralgia and post-herpetic pain, can also be treated by appropriate nerve blocks.

The sensory supply to the face and the anterior two-third of the scalp is provided by the trigeminal nerve. The posterior scalp is supplied by the greater and lesser cervical nerves from the cervical plexus. The anterior neck receives the transverse cutaneous nerve of the neck, which derives from the anterior primary rami of C2 and 3, as does the greater auricular nerve supplying the skin of the external ear and the skin below it. The posterior rami of C3, 4 and 5 supply the skin of the back of the neck.

The motor supply is from the facial nerve, which supplies the muscles of the face, and the trigeminal nerve which supplies the muscles of the mastication.

Trigeminal nerve block

Anatomy

The trigeminal nerve is the largest cranial nerve (Fig. 57:1). It is formed by the union of a sensory and a motor root. At the point of this union is the trigeminal (Gasserian) ganglion, which lies within the cranium in a depression close to the apex of the petrous part of the temporal bone. Through its three main branches it supplies the skin of the face and scalp, and the muscles of mastication (Fig. 57:2).

The three branches are:

1. The ophthalmic nerve, which leaves the cranium through the superior orbital fissure

2. The maxillary nerve, which leaves through the foramen rotundum

3. The mandibular nerve, which leaves through the foramen ovale

To block all three nerves with a single injection, the needle must reach the trigeminal ganglion by passing through the foramen ovale. Using a nerve stimulator, it is possible to identify the three main branches of the trigeminal nerve.

Because of the accuracy required in locating the foramen ovale, and the serious consequences of a misplaced injection, this block should only be done under radiographic control.

Fig. 57:1.
1. *Trigeminal nerve*
2. *Trigeminal (Gasserian) ganglion*
3. **Ophthalmic nerve**
4. *Nasociliary nerve*
5. *Supraorbital nerve*
6. *Lacrimal nerve*
7. *Frontal nerve*
8. *Supratrochlear nerve*
9. *Infratrochlear nerve*
10. **Maxillary nerve**
11. *Zygomatic nerve*
12. *Middle superior alveolar nerve*
13. *Posterior superior alveolar nerve*
14. *Anterior superior alveolar nerve*
15. *Infraorbital nerve*
16. **Mandibular nerve**
17. *Auriculotemporal nerve*
18. *Inferior alveolar nerve*
19. *Lingual nerve*
20. *Buccal nerve*
21. *Mental nerve*

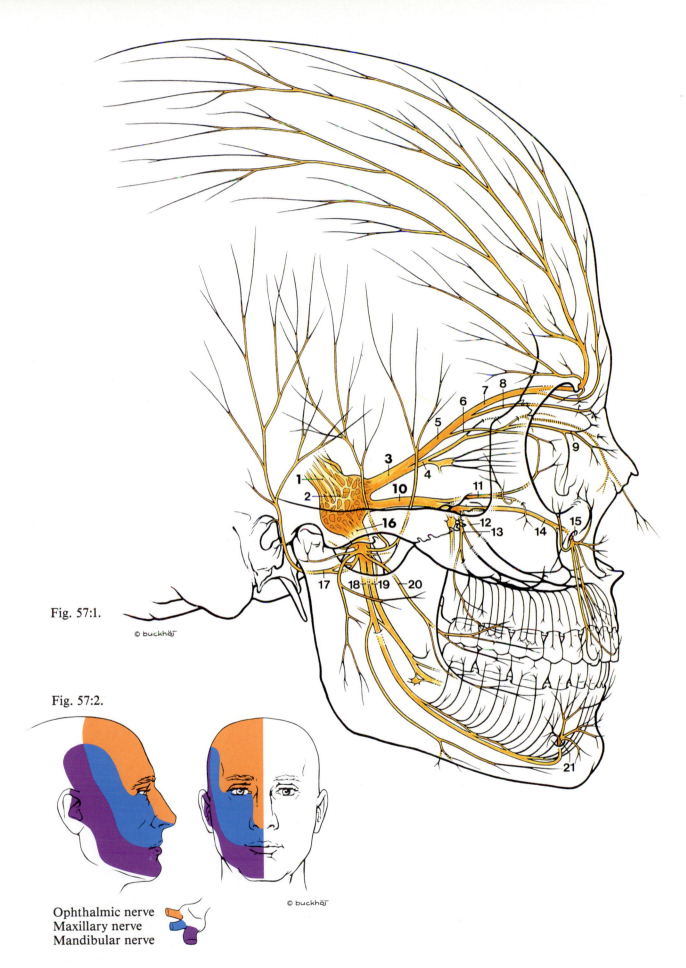

Fig. 57:1.

© buckhöj

Fig. 57:2.

© buckhöj

Ophthalmic nerve
Maxillary nerve
Mandibular nerve

Patient position

Supine with head in position to obtain a clear X-ray picture of the foramen ovale.

Landmarks

Fig. 59:3.
1. The pupil of the eye.
2. The midpoint of the zygoma.
3. Point 3 cm lateral to the lips, which should level with the pupil in the sagittal plane.

Needle insertion

A wheal is raised over (3) and the needle is inserted backwards and upwards in the direction of (1) and (2), so as to contact the greater wing of the sphenoid bone, anterior and superior to the foramen ovale. The direction is then altered using radiography until the tip just enters the foramen (Fig. 59:2 and 59:4). While the needle may elicit paraesthesia, a nerve stimulator can be used to identify the three main branches leaving the Gasserian ganglion. The ophthalmic branch is superior and medial, the mandibular is inferior and lateral, with the maxillary midway between. The needle should be carefully aspirated to eliminate an intravascular or subarachnoid position of the tip.

Drugs and dose

If a local anaesthetic is being used, 0.5-1 ml of 2% lidocaine or 0.5% bupivacaine or their equivalent (see p. 20) may be injected. However, it is more usual in the treatment of trigeminal neuralgia to perform a permanent neurolysis of one or more of the three nerves, depending upon the distribution of the pain. The choice of agent lies between alcohol 80% and phenol 5-10% in glycerine. 0.1 ml is injected and the effect assessed over several minutes before injecting a further 0.1 ml, continuing in this way until the required extent of nerve blockade is achieved.

Complications

1. Subarachnoid injection of local anaesthetic at the base of the brain can lead to unconsciousness and blockade of the ipsilateral cranial nerves.

2. Blockade of the ophthalmic nerve renders the eye analgesic and can lead to corneal ulceration.

Figs. 59:3.
1. The pupil of the eye.
2. The mid point of the zygoma.
3. Point 3 cm lateral to the lips, which should be level with (1) in the sagittal plane.

Fig. 59:2. Courtesy of Dr. G.L.M. Carmichael

Fig. 59:4. Courtesy of Dr. G.L.M. Carmichael

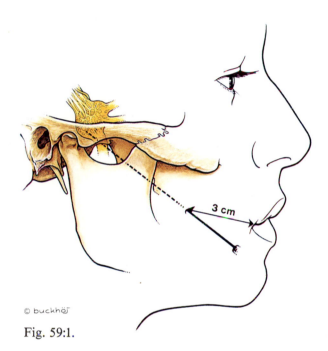

Fig. 59:1.

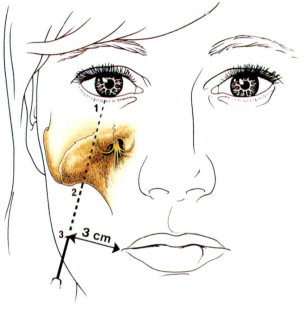

Fig. 59:3.

Fig. 59:2.

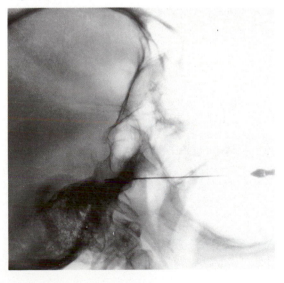

Fig. 59:4.

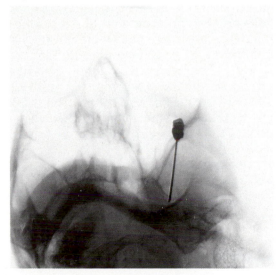

Ophthalmic nerve

Although the ophthalmic division of the trigeminal nerve can be permanently blocked close to the trigeminal ganglion, there are few indications for such a procedure, given the dangers of anaesthetising the eye with the possibility of corneal ulceration.

The branches of the ophthalmic nerve, however, which supply the skin of the upper eyelid, the forehead and the side of the nose, are readily blocked and this is of use in plastic surgery. The main branches are the nasociliary and the frontal nerves (Fig. 61:1).

Nasociliary nerve

The nasociliary nerve supplies the skin and mucous membrane of the nose, the cornea and the conjunctiva. Two internal nasal branches supply the mucous membrane of the anterior part of the nose, including the nasal septum. An external nasal branch supplies the skin of the lower part of the nose below the nasal bone. The long ciliary nerves supply the cornea and conjunctiva.

Patient position
Supine.

Landmarks
The orbit, the eyebrow and the medial palpebral fissure.

Needle insertion
The needle (23 gauge, 4 cm) is inserted perpendicularly backwards at the upper and medial part of the orbit, between the eyebrow and the palpebral fissure, closer to the former than the latter (Fig. 61:2). At a depth of about 1.5 cm the bone of the orbit will be contacted. If the bone is not contacted at this depth, the needle should be withdrawn and directed more medially until the medial wall of the orbit is felt at the depth of 1.5-2 cm. The optic nerve is 4 cm deep to the palpebral fissure.

Drugs and dose
After aspiration inject 2 ml of 1% lidocaine or 0.25% bupivacaine or their equivalent. (See p. 20).

Fig. 61:1. Courtesy of Astra
  1. Supraorbital nerve
  2. Frontal nerve
  3. Lacrimal nerve
  4. Nasociliary nerve
  5. Maxillary nerve
  6. Zygomatic nerve
  7. Infraorbital nerve
  8. Lateral branch of the frontal nerve
  9. Medial branch of the frontal nerve
  10. Supratrochlear nerve
  11. Infratrochlear nerve
  12. Nasopalatine nerve

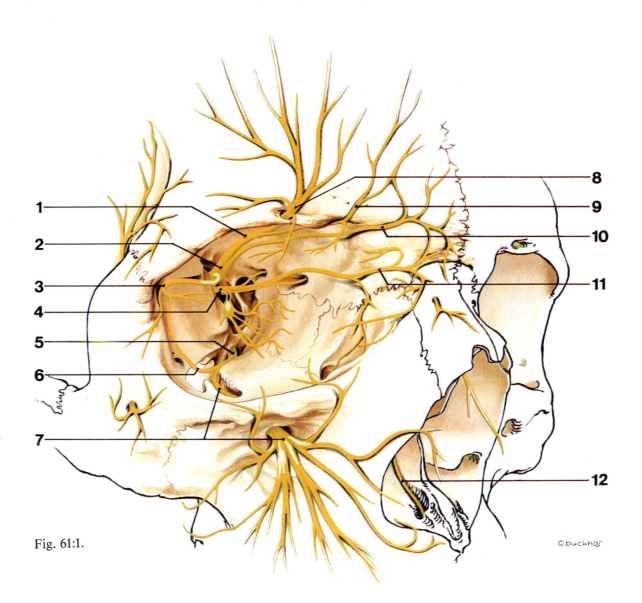

1
2
3
4
5
6
7

8
9
10
11

12

Fig. 61:1.

©buckhöj

Fig. 61:2.

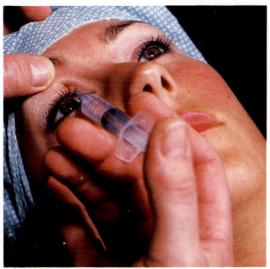

Frontal nerve

The supratrochlear nerve and the supraorbital nerves are the main branches of the frontal nerve, which runs along the superior wall of the orbit between the levator palpebrae superioris and the periosteum.

Supratrochlear nerve block

Anatomy
The supratrochlear nerve emerges from the orbit at its upper and medial part and runs upward under the frontal belly of the occipito-frontalis muscle to supply the skin of the medial aspect of the forehead. It also supplies the skin of the upper nose and sends branches to the conjunctivae and the upper eyelid.

Patient position
Supine.

Landmarks
The orbit and the eyebrow.

Needle insertion
The needle is inserted at the upper and medial part of the orbit. It is directed upwards and medially to contact the frontal bone just lateral to the root of the nose (Fig. 63:2).

Drugs and dose
After aspiration 2-3 ml of 1% lidocaine or 0.25% bupivacaine or their equivalent (see p. 20) is injected.

Supraorbital nerve block

Anatomy
The supraorbital nerve can leave the orbit through the supraorbital foramen before dividing into its medial and lateral branches. More frequently it divides before leaving the orbit, the lateral branch leaving through the foramen while the medial branch emerges 1 cm medial to the foramen (Fig. 63:1).

It supplies the upper eyelid and conjunctiva, before dividing and running upwards deep to the frontal belly of occipitofrontalis. After reaching the superficial fascia the two branches supply the skin of the scalp as far back as the lambdoid suture (Fig. 63:4).

Landmarks
The supraorbital foramen, which is palpable at the midpoint of the supraorbital margin of the orbit.

Needle insertion
While palpating the foramen the needle is inserted just under the eyebrow and directed upwards to lie close to the foramen (Figs. 63:3).

Drugs and dose
After aspiration 2-3 ml of 1% lidocaine or 0.25% bupivacaine or their equivalent is injected.

Superficial block of the supratrochlear and supraorbital nerves

The terminal cutaneous branches of these nerves, which supply the forehead and scalp, become superficial just above the eyebrow. They may be blocked by a subcutaneous infiltration in a horizontal line, 2 cm above the eyebrow from the lateral border of the orbit to the midline (Fig. 63:5).

Fig. 63:1. Courtesy of Astra.
1. *Lateral branch of the supraorbital nerve*
2. *Medial branch of the supraorbital nerve*
3. *Supratrochlear nerve*

Fig. 63:4. Courtesy of Astra.

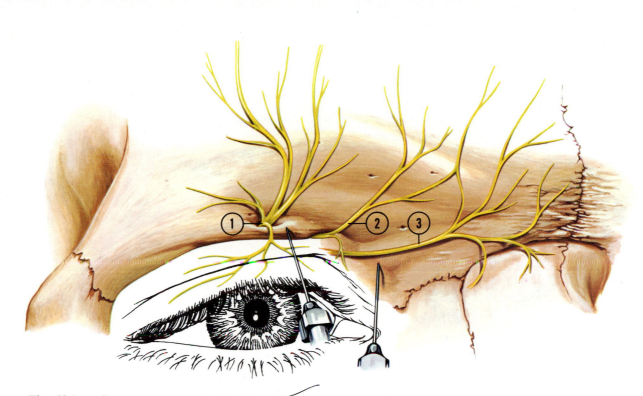

Fig. 63:1.

© buckhöj

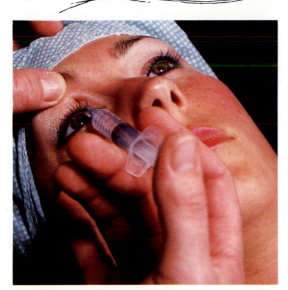

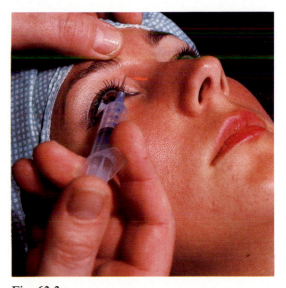

Fig. 63:2.
Fig. 63:4.

Fig. 63:3.
Fig. 63:5.

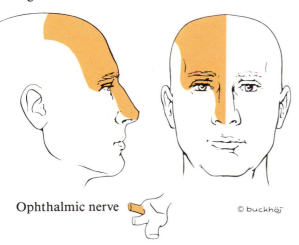

Ophthalmic nerve

© buckhöj

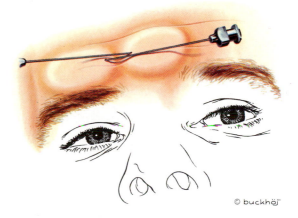

© buckhöj

63

Maxillary nerve block

While it is possible to block the terminal branches of the maxillary nerve, (i.e. the infraorbital, superior alveolar and palatine nerves), the maxillary nerve itself can be blocked more simply as it crosses the pterygopalatine fossa. This anaesthetises both the skin and the deep structures of the middle face, (Fig. 65:3) including the nasal cavity, the maxillary bone and sinus, the upper teeth, and the upper part of the mouth and the oral cavity.

Anatomy
The maxillary nerve leaves the cranium through the foramen rotundum, crosses the pterygopalatine fossa and enters the orbit through the inferior orbital fissure (Fig. 57:1), where it becomes the infraorbital nerve.

Branches of the maxillary nerve include the posterior, middle and anterior superior alveolar (dental) nerves, which supply the teeth in the upper jaw, together with the adjacent gums and mucous membrane. The anterior superior alveolar nerve also supplies the lateral wall and floor of the nasal cavity, together with part of the septum (Fig. 61:1).

Through its branches to the pterygopalatine ganglion, the maxillary nerve also supplies sensory fibres to the palate (both hard and soft), the tonsil and the lining of the posterior nasal cavity. The main nerves involved are the greater and lesser palatine nerves.

Patient position
Supine.

Landmarks
1. The zygoma
2. The anterior border of the ramus of the mandible, which is easily felt by opening and closing the mouth.

Needle insertion
At the junction of the zygoma and the anterior edge of the ramus, a 7 cm needle is inserted medially while inclined upwards and backwards. At about 4 cm the needle point will contact the sphenoid bone and paraesthesia may be elicited (Fig. 65:1).

Drugs and dose
After aspiration 4 ml of 1% lidocaine or 0.25% bupivacaine or their equivalent (see p. 20) is injected.

Infraorbital nerve block

Anatomy
The infraorbital nerve runs forward in the infraorbital groove and canal. It enters the face through the infraorbital foramen (Fig. 65:2). It lies under the levator labii superioris and its terminal branches supply the skin of the ala of the nose, the lower eyelid, the cheek and the upper lip. It also supplies the mucous membrane on the inside of the cheek and upper lip.

Landmarks
1. The lower border of the orbit.
2. The infraorbital foramen.

Needle insertion.
This may be through the skin of the face or through the mouth.

The **transcutaneous** approach (Fig. 65:4) is made by inserting the needle at the midpoint of the lower border of the orbit, 1 cm below that border. The infraorbital foramen can usually be palpated at this point. The needle is directed upwards to be close to the foramen and paraesthesia may be elicited.

In the **transoral approach** (Fig. 65:5) the needle is inserted through the superior buccal sulcus and directed upwards to the infraorbital foramen, which is being palpated with the other hand. The needle tip can be felt as it approaches the foramen.

Because of the retrograde spread through the infraorbital foramen the incisor, canine and premolar teeth and the surrounding gums will also be anaesthetised (supplied by the anterior alveolar nerves).

Drugs and dose
After aspiration 2-3 ml of 1% lidocaine or 0.25% bupivacaine or their equivalent (see p. 20) is injected.

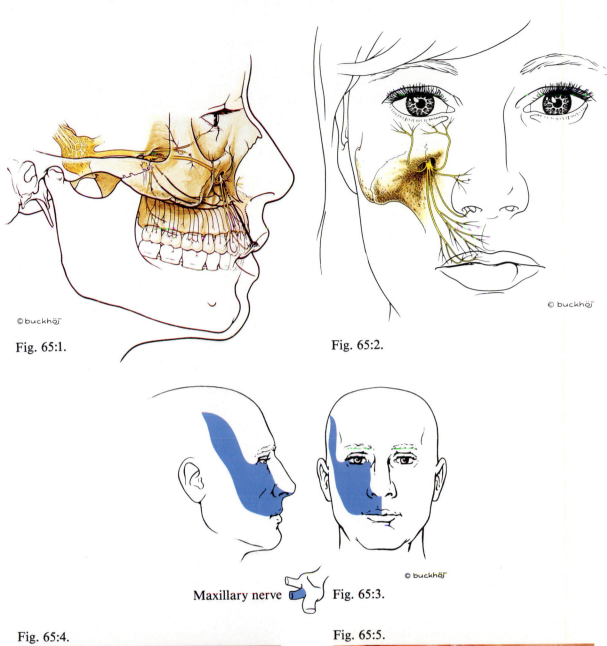

Fig. 65:1.

Fig. 65:2.

Maxillary nerve  Fig. 65:3.

Fig. 65:4.

Fig. 65:5.

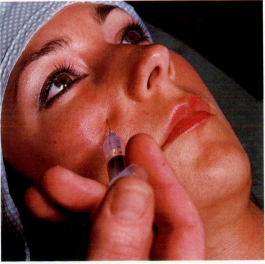

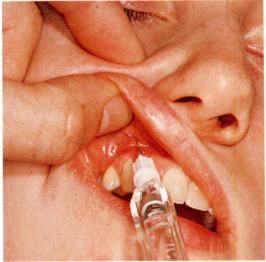

Mandibular nerve block

While it is more usual to block the terminal branches of the mandibular nerve, the main nerve can be blocked as it leaves the foramen ovale.

This will anaesthetise the lower jaw and the skin and tissues of the lower face and can be used as an adjunct to general anaesthesia in major operations on the jaw.

Anatomy

The mandibular nerve is the largest branch of the trigeminal nerve (Fig. 67:1). It is both sensory and motor. The sensory nerves supply the skin over the lower jaw, the posterior part of the face and the temporal region, (Fig. 67:2) the mucous membrane of the lower lip and the floor of the mouth, and the lower teeth and gums. The motor branches supply the muscles of mastication.

The large sensory root leaves the cranium through the foramen ovale, where it is joined by the motor root. After giving off a meningeal branch and the nerve to the medial pterygoid muscle, the mandibular nerve divides into an anterior and a posterior trunk. The sensory fibres of the anterior trunk run in the **buccal nerve**, which is distributed with branches of the facial nerve. It supplies the skin and mucous membrane on either side of the buccinator muscle and the posterior part of the buccal surface of the gum of the lower jaw. The motor fibres supply the masseter and temporalis muscles.

The posterior trunk divides into three branches, the auriculotemporal, the lingual and the inferior alveolar nerves. The **auriculotemporal nerve** supplies the skin over the temporal region, the skin anterior to the ear (including the tragus) and the external auditory meatus (including the tympanic membrane). The **lingual nerve** supplies the mucous membrane of the floor of the mouth and the anterior two-thirds of the tongue, in addition to the lingual surface of the lower gums. The **inferior alveolar nerve** enters the mandibular foramen and runs in the mandibular canal supplying the lower teeth. At the mental foramen it gives off a lateral branch, the **mental nerve**, which supplies the skin over the anterior jaw and the lower lip (both mucous membrane and skin).

Patient position

Supine with head in neutral position, mouth closed.

Landmarks

1. The zygomatic arch
2. The condyle of the mandible
3. The coronoid process of the mandible

2 and 3 are identified by opening and closing the mouth.

Needle insertion

A wheal is raised 0.5 cm below the zygomatic arch midway between the coronoid process and the condyle of the mandible. The needle is inserted at right angles to the skin until it contacts the pterygoid plate at a depth of 3-4 cm (Figs. 67:3 and 67:4). It is withdrawn a few millimetres and redirected 20° posteriorly until a paraesthesia is elicited.

Drugs and dose

5 ml of 2% lidocaine or 0.5% bupivacaine or their equivalent (see p. 20).

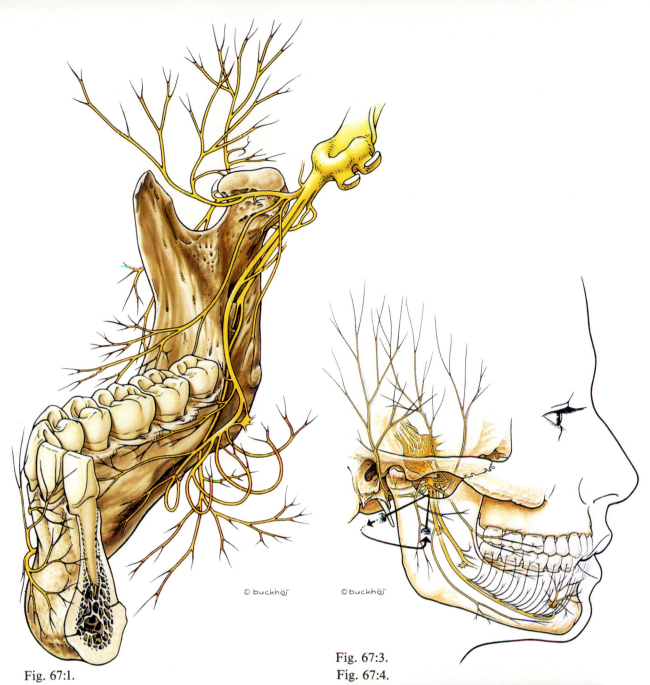

Fig. 67:1.

Fig. 67:2.

Fig. 67:3.

Fig. 67:4.

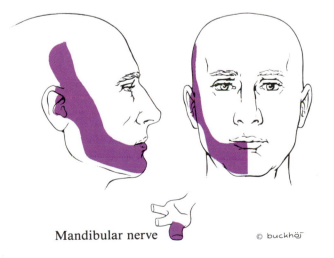

Mandibular nerve

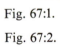

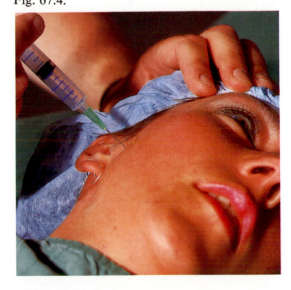

Inferior alveolar nerve block

This is commonly used in dentistry and is frequently (incorrectly) called a mandibular block. It is also useful in oral surgery to supplement general anaesthesia and to provide postoperative analgesia.

Anatomy

The **inferior alveolar nerve** enters the mandibular foramen and runs in the mandibular canal supplying the lower teeth. At the mental foramen it gives off a lateral branch, the **mental nerve**, which supplies the skin over the anterior jaw and the lower lip (both mucous membrane and skin).

Patient position

Sitting or supine, mouth widely open.

Landmarks

1. The molar teeth
2. The anterior border of the ramus of the mandible

Needle insertion

With the forefinger of the non-dominant hand on the ramus of the mandible the needle is inserted 1 cm above the occlusal surfaces of the molar teeth. The syringe is directed from the premolar teeth of the **opposite** side, so as to contact the medial side of the ramus. After the initial insertion, the patient should close the mouth a little to relax the pterygoid muscle (Fig. 69:1 and 3). Keeping the syringe parallel to the teeth the needle is advanced 1.5-2 cm, keeping the point in contact with the bone (Fig. 69:2). At the midsection of the ramus, resistance will be met. The needle is withdrawn 1-2 mm and the injection made (Fig. 69:4).

Drugs and dose

1.5-2 ml of 2% lidocaine with adrenaline 1:80.000 or 3% prilocaine with felypressin (Octapressin) 0.03 IU/ml. This is usually administered with a dental cartridge syringe.

Lingual nerve block

This is usually done in conjunction with inferior alveolar nerve block. After blocking that nerve, the needle is withdrawn 5 mm and a further 0.5 ml of local anaesthetic injected (Fig. 69:5). It anaesthetises the floor of the mouth, the anterior two-thirds of the tongue and the lingual surface of the lower gums.

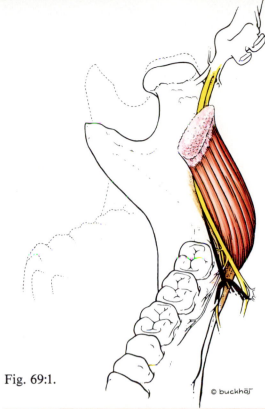

Fig. 69:1.

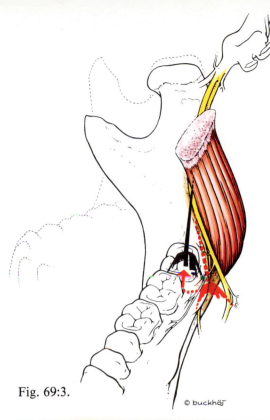

Fig. 69:3.

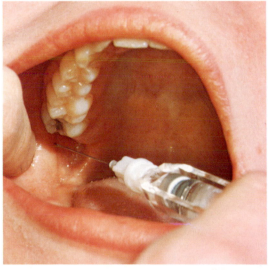

Fig. 69:2.

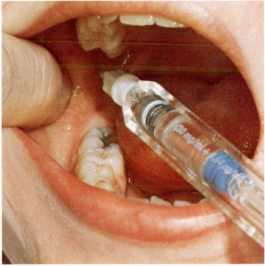

Fig. 69:4.

Fig. 69:5.

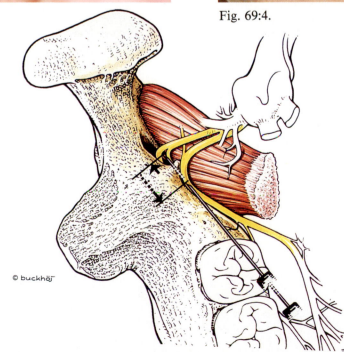

Mental nerve block

Anatomy
The mental nerve supplies the lower lip and the skin of the anterior part of the jaw. It is blocked as it emerges from the mental foramen (Fig. 71:1). Because some of the injected drug will enter the foramen and pass in a retrograde fashion to reach the inferior alveolar nerve, a mental block will also anaesthetise the incisor, the canine and the premolar teeth. It is not recommended that the mental foramen is entered as this can cause damage to the nerve with prolonged analgesia of the lower lip. The local anaesthetic should be deposited around the outside of the mental foramen. Although this can be done transcutaneously, it is more convenient to do it intraorally.

Intraoral approach

Patient position
Mouth open and lower lip retracted.

Landmarks
The mental foramen is palpated just posterior to the first premolar tooth 1 cm below the gum margin.

Needle insertion
The needle is inserted 1 cm below the first premolar directed backwards and medially to contact the bone near the foramen but not to enter it (Fig. 71:2).

Transcutaneous approach
The mental foramen is palpated through the skin and a needle is directed upwards, medially and backwards to contact the mandible at the foramen (Fig. 71:3).

Drugs and dose
1-1.5 ml of 2% lidocaine with adrenaline 1:80.000 or 3% prilocaine with felypressin (Octapressin) 0.03 IU/ml.

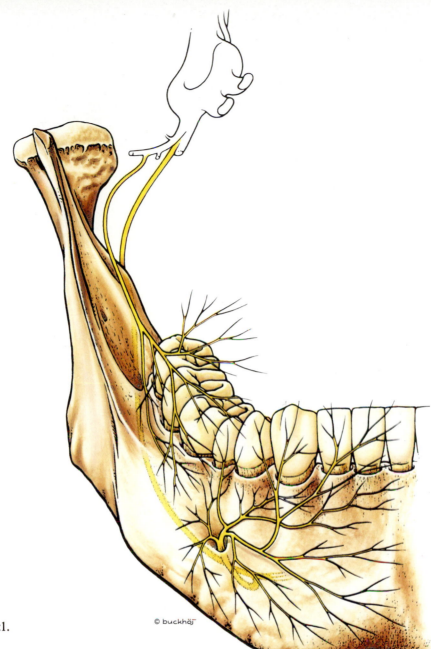

Fig. 71:1.

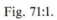

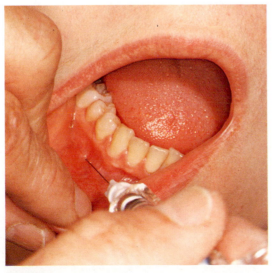

Fig. 71:2.

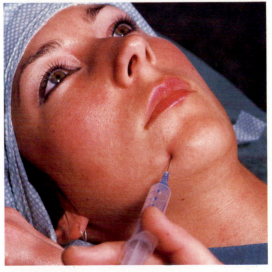

Fig. 71:3.

Superior laryngeal nerve block

Anatomy
An aid to anaesthetising the larynx is by superior laryngeal nerve block (Fig. 73:1). This nerve, a branch of the vagus nerve, runs behind the greater cornu of the hyoid bone where it divides into the internal and external laryngeal nerves. The former pierces the thyrohyoid membrane midway between the thyroid and hyoid bones to provide the sensory innervation to the larynx and the lower pharynx including the epiglottis. The external laryngeal nerve supplies the cricothyroid muscle and the inferior constrictor of the pharynx.

For topical anaesthesia of the larynx see page 34.

Patient position
Supine or sitting up.

Landmarks
1. Thyroid cartilage
2. Hyoid bone (greater cornuae)

Needle insertion
Using a median approach (Figs. 73:2 and 73:3), a needle is inserted at the upper border of the thyroid bone and directed laterally and superiorly towards the posterior part of the greater cornu of the hyoid bone using the index finger to guide it.

Alternatively, using a lateral approach two injections can be made, one on each side, just inferior to the posterior part of the greater cornuae.

Drug and dose
2-3 ml of 2% lidocaine or its equivalent (see p. 21) will block each nerve. The injection is then repeated on the opposite side. This will render the larynx anaesthetic without gross impairment of the muscles of the larynx which are supplied by the recurrent laryngeal nerves, and are unaffected by this block.

Fig. 73:1.
1. Superior laryngeal nerve
2. Internal laryngeal nerve

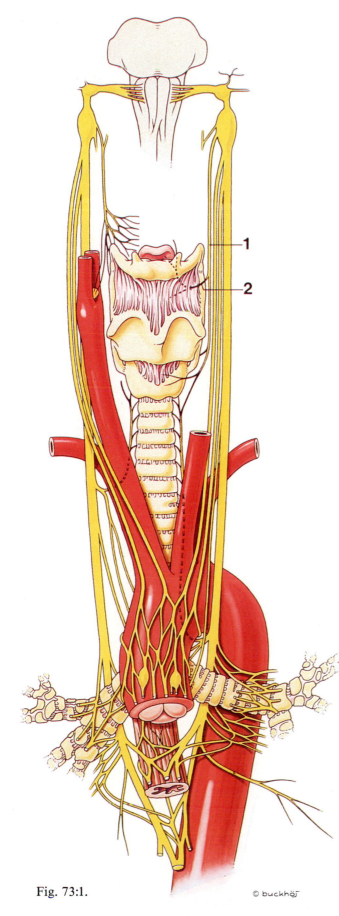

Fig. 73:1.

© buckhöj

1
2

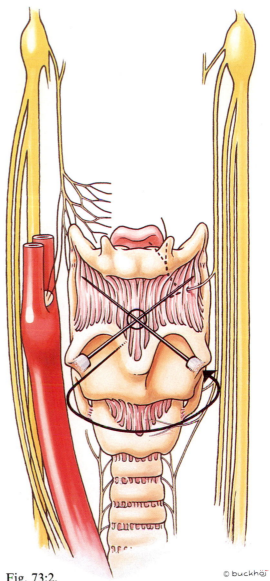

Fig. 73:2.

© buckhöj

Fig. 73:3.

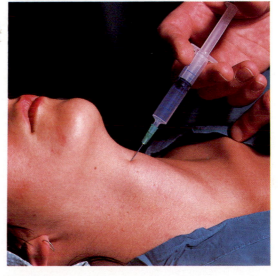

73

Cervical plexus block

Anatomy
Like other spinal nerves, the cervical spinal nerves on leaving the spinal canal (posterior to the vertebral artery) divide into dorsal and ventral rami (Fig. 75:2). The dorsal rami curve backwards and supply the muscles of the back of the head and neck and innervate the skin from the vertex to the shoulders.

The ventral rami of the upper four cervical nerves form the cervical plexus (the lower four join the brachial plexus). This plexus innervates the skin of the front of the neck, the shoulders and the upper chest, together with the neck muscles. The plexus lies over the upper four cervical vertebrae, deep to the internal jugular vein and the sternomastoid muscle, and anterior to the scalenus medius and levator scapulae (Fig. 75:1). There is considerable intercommunication between adjacent nerves.

The branches of the plexus are divided into superficial and deep. The superficial branches pierce the cervical fascia just posterior to the sternomastoid and supply the skin of the side of the face and the neck. The deep branches are mostly motor nerves to the muscles of the neck and the phrenic nerve. Blockade of the superficial branches is easily performed but will only anaesthetise the skin. Blockade of the individual cervical nerves as they leave the vertebrae will also affect the muscles (including the diaphragm) and other deep structures. Although each nerve may be blocked individually, it is much easier to make a single injection at C3. Because local anaesthetic spreads paravertebrally quite readily, C2 and C4 will be blocked together with C3.

Indications for cervical plexus block are:

1. Superficial operations on the neck and shoulders
2. Operations on the thyroid gland
3. Pain therapy

Patient position
Supine with head extended and turned to opposite side.

Landmarks
Fig. 75:3.
1. The mastoid process
2. The transverse process of C6 (Chassaignac's tubercle), which is the most prominent of the transverse processes and is at the level of the cricoid cartilage
3. The sternomastoid muscle

Joining 1 and 2 gives the line for identifying the individual vertebrae, the transverse processes of which lie just posterior to the line.

Fig. 75:1. Courtesy of Astra.
1. Mastoid process
2. Sternomastoid muscle
3. Transverse process of C6

Fig. 75:2.
1. Posterior primary ramus
2. Anterior primary ramus
3. Grey ramus communicans
4. Vertebral artery
5. Superior cervical ganglion

Fig. 75:3.
1. Scalenus anterior muscle
2. Scalenus medius muscle
3. Sympathetic chain
4. Spinal root C1

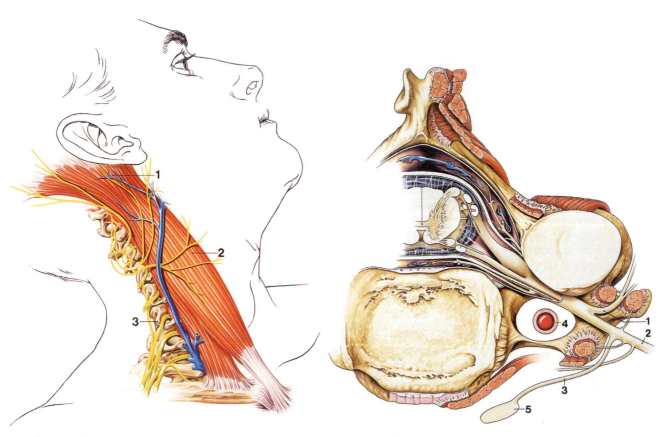

Fig. 75:1.

© buckhöj

Fig. 75:2.

© buckhöj

Fig. 75:3.

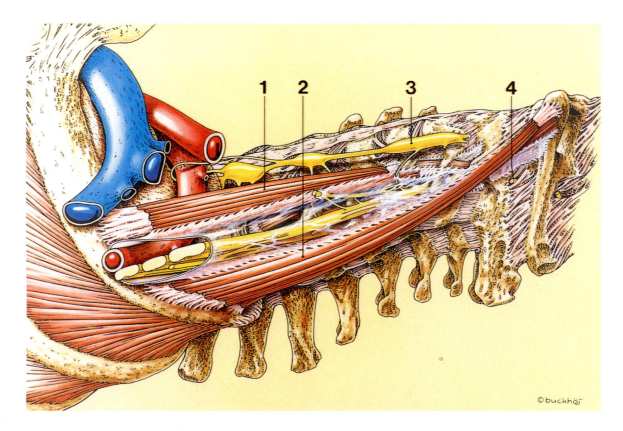

© buckhöj

Needle insertion

For a superficial block, the subcutaneous tissues are infiltrated in the line of the posterior border of the sternomastoid, the central point of the infiltration being at C3-4 (Fig. 77:1). This anaesthetises the skin only, in the distribution of the lesser occipital, the greater auricular, the transverse cutaneous nerve of the neck and the supraclavicular nerves.

For a deep block, the needle is directed towards the transverse processes of C3, at right angles to the skin and pointing slightly caudad. It is advanced 1.5-3 cm so as to contact bone or elicit a paraesthesia. The needle hub should be carefully examined for escape of blood or cerebrospinal fluid (Fig. 77:2 and 77:4).

Drugs and dose

For a superficial block, 10 ml of 1% lidocaine or 0.25% bupivacaine on each side.

For a deep block, 10 ml of 2% lidocaine or 0.5% bupivacaine (with epinephrine 1:200.000 for a prolonged block). If a bilateral block is being done, the concentration should be reduced to 1%, to lessen the risk of bilateral phrenic paralysis.

Complications

1. Subarachnoid injection leading to a high spinal block. The patient will usually become unconscious and may stop breathing. Severe hypotension may also occur. Treatment consists of artificial ventilation and a vasopressor to support the circulation.

2. Epidural injection which will cause anaesthesia in the upper limbs and thorax. Unlike a subarachnoid injection, the local anaesthetic cannot spread into the cranium.

3. Intravenous injection leading to generalised toxicity.

4. Intra-arterial injection due to the close proximity of the vertebral artery. As the local anaesthetic drug will go direct to the brain, very small quantities can cause convulsions and apnoea.

5. Phrenic nerve paralysis which may lead to respiratory difficulties, particularly if there is pre-existing lung disease.

6. Anaesthesia of other nerves in the neck such as the vagus, glossopharyngeal and cervical sympathetic chain. This can cause hoarseness (due to recurrent laryngeal nerve block), difficulty in swallowing, Horner's syndrome, etc.

Suggested further reading

Evers, H. & Haegerstam, G (1981) Handbook of Dental Local Anaesthesia, Schultz, Copenhagen.
Gautier-Lafaye, P. (1985) Laco-regional anaesthesia for the head & neck. In Précis d'Anesthésie Loco-Régionals. Masson, Paris, p. 47.

Fig. 77:1, 2 and 3. Courtesy of Astra.

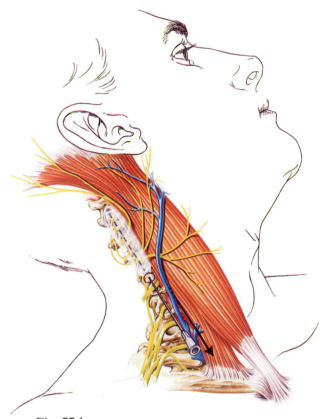

Fig. 77:1.

Fig. 77:2.

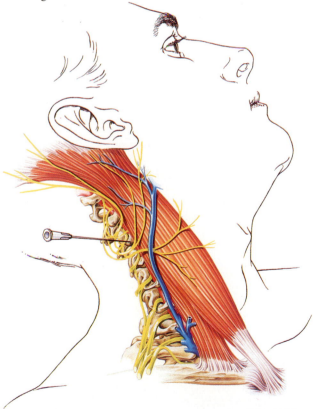

© buckhöj

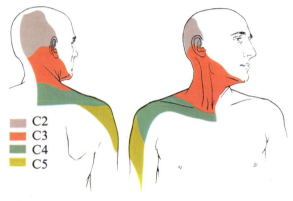

Fig. 77:3.

© buckhöj

C2
C3
C4
C5

Fig. 77:4.

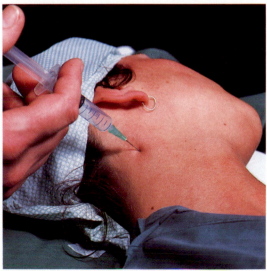

Local anaesthesia in ophthalmology

Anatomy

The somatic sensory nerves to the eyeball run in the long ciliary nerves which derive from the nasociliary nerve, a branch of the ophthalmic nerve (Fig. 79:2). The sensory nerves to the upper eyelid and adjacent skin also come from the ophthalmic division of the trigeminal nerve (Fig. 57:2), while the lower lid is supplied by the maxillary division (see p. 64).

The motor nerves to the extrinsic muscles of the eyeball come from the superior and inferior rami of the oculomotor nerve. The orbicularis occuli muscle is supplied by branches of the facial nerve.

The sympathetic fibres, which are sensory, motor and vasomotor, come from the superior cervical ganglia and although they pass through the ciliary ganglion, they do not synapse there (Figs. 79:1). They reach the eyeball through the short ciliary nerves. The motor fibres supply the dilator pupillae muscle.

The parasympathetic supply comes from the oculomotor nerve and the fibres enter the ciliary ganglion, where they synapse. The postganglionic fibres run in the short ciliary nerves and supply the constrictor pupillae muscle (Fig. 79:1).

The eyeball, including its intrinsic and extrinsic muscles, can be blocked by injecting local anaesthetic into the cone formed by the extrinsic muscles, close to the ciliary ganglion i.e. a retrobulbar injection.

Principles

To perform painless surgery in ophthalmological practice, it is necessary to consider the eye and its surrounding tissues as six separate components, namely:

1. The cornea, which is easily anaesthetised by topical local anaesthesia

2. The conjunctiva, which is more difficult to anaesthetise topically but can additionally be anaesthetised by local infiltration or nerve blockade

3. The eyeball itself (together with the intrinsic and extrinsic muscles), which is anaesthetised by a retrobulbar injection

4. The eyelids and the adjacent skin, which are anaesthetised by local infiltration

5. The tear sac and tear ducts, which can be locally infiltrated but will also require anaesthesia of the nasal mucosal membrane

6. The orbicularis oculi muscles, which must be paralysed during intraocular surgery. It is extremely important to avoid blepharospasm during open surgery of the eyeball as it not only seriously hinders access for the surgeon, but can also discharge the contents of the eye. Thus it is necessary to paralyse this muscle by blocking the branches of the facial nerve which supply it.

Patient management

It is very important to avoid restlessness of the patient, which can be both inconvenient and dangerous.

Good rapport with the patient is essential to avoid undue nervousness and anxiety. Some form of sedation (see p. 14) may be required, especially when open operations of the eyeball are to be performed. However, older patients who are unsedated, are generally easier to deal with than those who are sedated.

Fig. 79:1.
1. Stellate ganglion
2. Middle cervical ganglion
3. Superior cervical ganglion
4. *Plexus internal carotid*
5. Trigeminal nerve (V)
6. Trigeminal (seminular) ganglion
7. Oculomotor nerve (III)
8. Nasociliary nerve
9. Long ciliary nerves
10. Ciliary ganglion
11. Cornea
12. Sphincter pupillae muscle
13. Iris
14. Dilatator pupillae muscle
15. Vas
16. Ciliaris muscle
17. Ciliary body

Fig. 79:2. Courtesy of Astra.
1. Inferior ophthalmic vein
2. Inferior oblique muscle
3. Lateral rectus muscle
4. Inferior rectus muscle
5. Ciliary ganglion

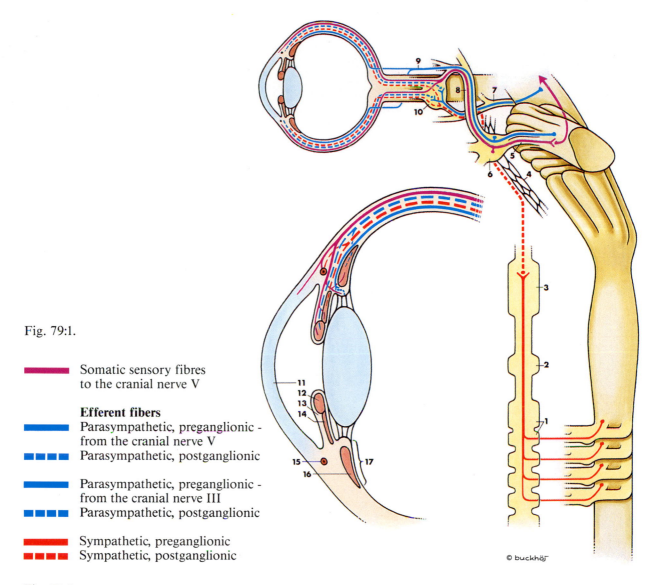

Fig. 79:1.

Fig. 79:2.

Somatic sensory fibres
to the cranial nerve V

Efferent fibers
Parasympathetic, preganglionic -
from the cranial nerve V
Parasympathetic, postganglionic

Parasympathetic, preganglionic -
from the cranial nerve III
Parasympathetic, postganglionic

Sympathetic, preganglionic
Sympathetic, postganglionic

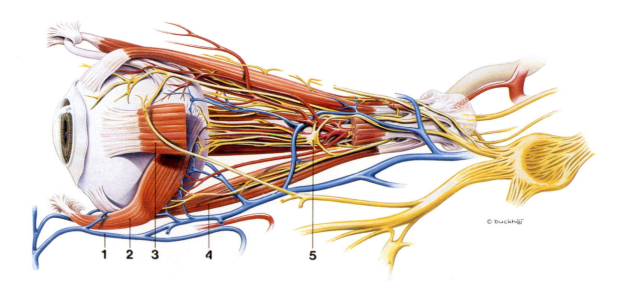

Topical anaesthesia

This can be used for virtually all simple ocular manoeuvres and should precede any injection of the conjunctiva. The eye cannot retain more than about 1 drop of fluid, any excess running out onto the face. Thus only a limited amount of local anaesthetic can be absorbed after each instillation, regardless of the amount instilled. The cornea is usually anaesthetised with a single instillation, but the patient should be warned that all local anaesthetics sting a little on their first instillation, and this may last 15-30 s. If a second or subsequent application does not sting, it may be assumed that the cornea is anaesthetised.

The conjunctiva is more resistant because of its much greater blood supply and it will usually require repeated instillations every 30-45 s. The anaesthesia does not last long and further drops may be required during surgery. Even with a retrobulbar injection which totally anaesthetises the eyeball, the conjunctiva may require further topical applications if it is to be stitched at the end of surgery. Likewise, the removal of stitches will need several repeated drops.

Drugs and dose

A wide variety of local anaesthetics is available, including lidocaine 4%, tetracaine (Amethocaine) 1%, oxybuprocaine (Benoxinate) 0.2% and cocaine 5%. Oxybuprocaine precipitates when added to fluorescein.

Figs. 81:1 and 2. Courtesy of Astra.

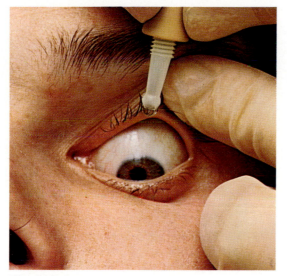

Fig. 81:1.

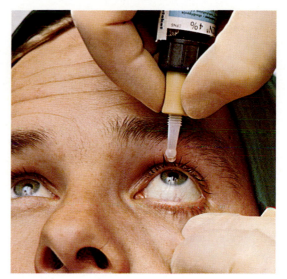

Fig. 81:2.

Local infiltration

This can be used for operations on the eyelids (and/or the adjacent skin), the conjunctiva and the tear sac and ducts.

Eyelids

To anaesthetise the eyelids, topical local anaesthetic is first applied to the conjunctiva. The eyelid (upper or lower) is everted and a fine needle inserted into the conjunctiva at the lateral part of the lid and advanced along its whole length, injecting as the needle is moving (Fig. 83:1). The needle is withdrawn back to its point of insertion, and while still in the subconjunctival tissue, the eyelid is inverted to its normal position. The needle is then turned outwards and pushed through the orbital septum to enter the subcutaneous aspect of the eyelid. Local anaesthetic is then deposited along the length of the lid subcutaneously.

This simple block will allow all types of reconstructive surgery on the eyelid. It should be remembered that the infiltration will swell the lid and it may be difficult to locate, say, a tarsal cyst unless it has been identified and marked before the injection.

Drugs and dose
4-5 ml of 0.5 or 1% lidocaine or its equivalent (see p. 20).

Conjunctiva

Infiltration of the conjunctiva (after initial topical anaesthesia) will allow operations such as cryocoagulation of the retina. The anaesthetic is deposited just behind the insertion of the rectus muscle, i.e. where the retina ends.

Drugs and dose
1-3 ml of 0.5% lidocaine or its equivalent (see p. 20).

Tear sac and tear ducts

A needle is inserted 0.5 cm above the medial canthus and directed backwards and medially until it contacts the orbital septum. 0.5 ml of local anaesthetic is injected and the needle redirected more medially to contact the medial wall of the orbit, above the medial palpebral ligament, where a further 0.5 ml is injected. These injections are repeated in relation to the lower eyelid, the needle penetrating the orbital septum just below the medial palpebral ligament (Fig. 83:2).

The nasal mucous membrane is anaesthetised by spraying the nose and applying gauze soaked in local anaesthetic (see p. 36).

Drugs and dose
2 ml of 0.5% lidocaine or its equivalent for the injection, and 5 ml of 4% lidocaine for the nasal mucous membrane. Operative bleeding will be greatly reduced by adding epinephrine, 1:200.000, to the injection and 0.25 ml of 1:1.000 (250 µg) to the topical solution.

Figs. 83:1 and 2. Courtesy of Astra.

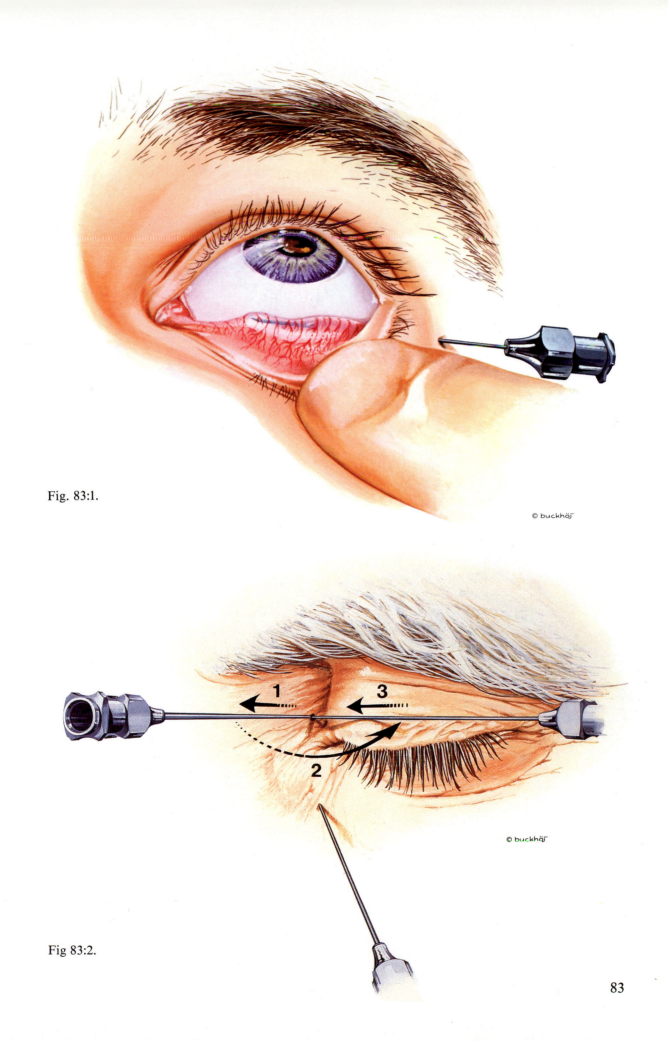

Fig. 83:1.

© buckhöj

Fig 83:2.

© buckhöj

83

Retrobulbar injection

This allows all forms of operation upon the eyeball. However, if the conjunctiva requires stitching at the end of surgery, further topical application or local infiltration may be required. The object of a retrobulbar injection is to deposit local anaesthetic within the cone formed by the extra-ocular muscles, as close as possible to the ciliary ganglion (Fig. 85:1). This effectively denervates the eyeball, leaving it paralysed with a dilated pupil and reduced intra-ocular pressure. There is usually a degree of exophthalmos from the volume of fluid injected.

Patient position
Supine. Patient should look upwards and towards the non-operated side.

Landmarks
1. The lateral canthus
2. The inferolateral angle of the orbit

Needle insertion
A 3.5-cm needle is used. It is inserted through the skin 1 cm below and 0.5 cm medial to the lateral canthus at the level of the inferolateral angle of the orbit (Figs. 85:2 and 85:3). It is directed medially, superiorly and posteriorly towards the apex of the orbit. The eyeball may be gently retracted medially with the forefinger of the non-dominant hand. To push away structures, particularly blood vessels, in the path of the needle, local anaesthetic should be injected slowly but continuously as the needle is advanced. The orbital septum of the lower eyelid will be felt as it is pierced. The needle is inserted to its full 3.5 cm (Fig. 85:4). After careful aspiration, the main injection is made. 5 min should be allowed for the block to become fully effective. The application of a tight pressure dressing to the eye aids diffusion of the local anaesthetic.

Drugs and dose
To allow the maximum effect from a small volume of local anaesthetic, it is necessary to use higher concentrations than in the other ophthalmological blocks. 2-3 ml of 2% lidocaine or its equivalent (see p. 21) is sufficient to anaesthetise the eye. The use of a larger volume (10-12 ml) has the advantage of spreading the drug to anaesthetise both the eye and the orbicularis oculi muscle allowing intra-ocular surgery with a single injection.

Complications
1. Retrobulbar haematoma. This will be diagnosed by increasing exophthalmos in the first minutes after injection. If it occurs, the operation should be abandoned otherwise the increased pressure on the eyeball may discharge its contents when it is opened.
2. Transfixion of the eyeball by the needle if the direction is too medial.
3. Intra-arterial injection. If local anaesthetic is injected into an artery, it can travel in a retrograde fashion and reach the internal carotid artery and thus gain direct access to the brain. In this way the classical signs and symptoms of overdosage (see p. 22) can occur even with small amounts of drug.
4. Subarachnoid injection. A dural cuff containing cerebrospinal fluid surrounds the optic nerves and may be entered by the needle. Local anaesthetic can then reach the optic chiasma and the adjacent structures, leading to blindness in the contralateral eye, convulsions, apnoea and unconsciousness. Provided vital functions are supported, all these effects will disappear once the local anaesthetic has been absorbed.

Injection into the optic nerve covrings requires a relatively high pressure and the injection should be stopped if resistance is encountered. Before attaching the syringe, small movements of the needle will cause the eyeball to move if the nerve has been entered.

Figs. 85:1 and 2. Courtesy of Astra.

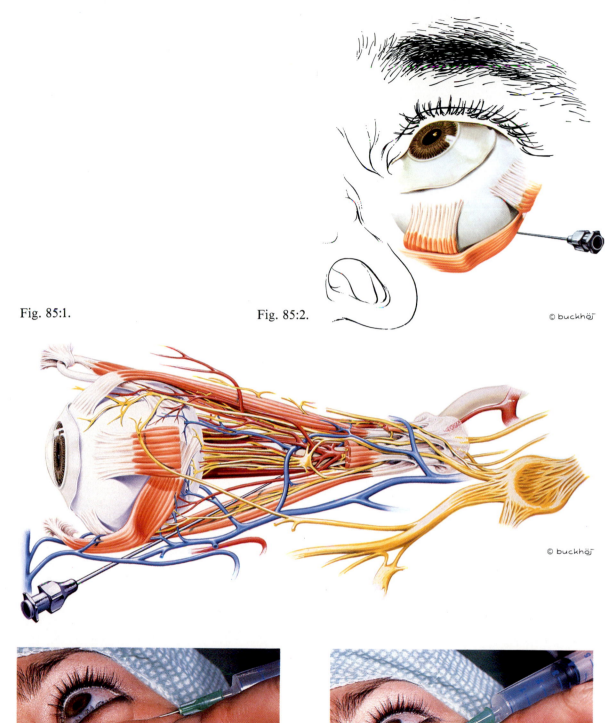

Fig. 85:1.

Fig. 85:2.

© buckhöj

© buckhöj

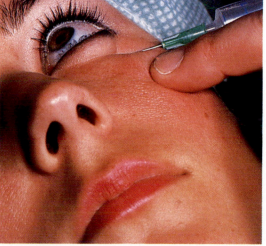

Fig. 85:3.

Fig. 85:4.

Motor blockade of the orbicularis oculi muscle

It is important to paralyse the orbicularis oculi muscle if intra-ocular surgery is being performed to prevent blepharospasm, which impedes surgical access and may discharge the contents of the eye.

Anatomy

The orbicularis oculi muscle is supplied by the temporal and zygomatic branches of the facial nerve. These cross the zygomatic bone en route to the muscle and can be blocked by infiltration of the facial tissues in this area (technique of Van Lint).

The facial nerve itself enters the face through the stylomastoid foramen and crosses the condyle of the mandible in the substance of the parotid gland, where it can be blocked by the O'Brien method. It supplies all the facial muscles.

Van Lint technique

Landmarks
1. The zygomatic bone and arch
2. The lateral canthus

Needle insertion
The needle is inserted over the zygomatic bone 2-3 cm below the lateral canthus (Fig. 87:1). The needle should contact the zygomatic bone where 2 ml of local anaesthetic is injected. It is then directed upwards and laterally to pass 1 cm behind the lateral canthus, within the deep tissues. As it is withdrawn, 2-3 ml of local anaesthetic is injected. On reaching the subcutaneous tissue, the needle is redirected at right angles parallel to the inferior margin of the orbit, and a further 2-3 ml injected on withdrawal. Some authorities also inject along the superior margin of the orbit.

Drugs and dose
6-8 ml of lidocaine 1% or its equivalent (see p. 20).

O'Brien technique

Landmarks
1. The condyle of the mandible
2. The tragus of the ear
3. The zygomatic arch

Needle insertion
The needle is inserted perpendicularly to the skin towards the mandibular condyle just in front of the tragus (Fig. 87:2). After contacting the condyle, the needle is slowly withdrawn as 2-4 ml of local anaesthetic is injected. This should block the nerve but the blockade may be reinforced by further injections through the same puncture site, the needle being directed first vertically, then towards the anterior part of the zygomatic arch and finally towards the middle of the arch. After each advancement 2-4 ml is injected as the needle is withdrawn.

Drugs and dose
8-16 ml of 1% lidocaine or its equivalent (see p. 20).

As previously mentioned (p. 84) some authorities use a large volume retrobulbar block alone, which will anaesthetise the eyeball and the orbicularis oculi. Motor paralysis of the muscle is easily tested and should be confirmed before starting surgery.

Fig. 87:1. Courtesy of Astra.

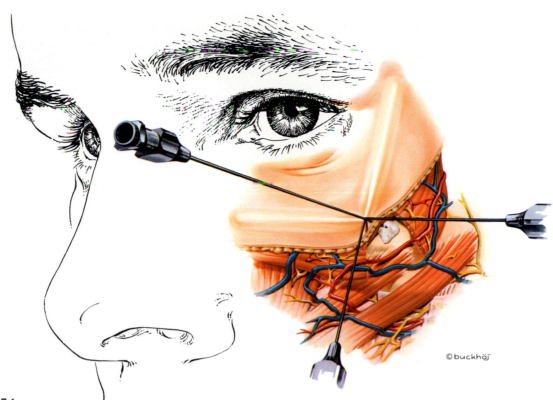

Fig. 87:1.

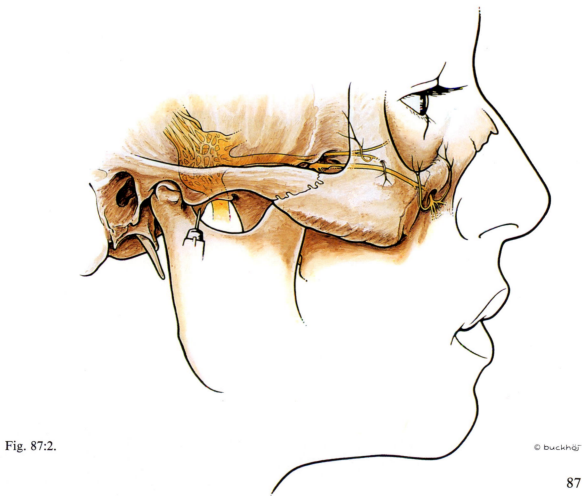

Fig. 87:2.

Other nerve blocks

Blockade of the terminal branches of the ophthalmic and maxillary divisions of the trigeminal nerve have been described on p. 60-65. They can be used for operations on and around the eyelids and may be preferred to local infiltration if the swelling this causes is to be avoided.

Suggested further reading

Feitl, M.E. & Krupin, T. (1988) Neural blockade for ophthalmologic surgery. In Neural Blockade eds Cousins M.J. & Bridenbaugh, P.O. Lippincott, Philadelphia, p. 577.

Upper and lower limb

Upper limb

Brachial plexus block

Anatomy
The brachial plexus is formed principally from the arterior primary rami of the C5, C6, C7, C8 and T1 spinal nerves. It runs from the vertebral column, passes between clavicle and first rib and enters the upper limb in the axilla before dividing into its four main terminal branches, the median, the radial, the ulnar and the musculo-cutaneous nerves.

The plexus may be blocked with local anaesthetic at any point in its course from the neck to the axilla. The three commonest approaches are the interscalene, the supraclavicular and the axillary. Because the surrounding connective tissue forms a tube, the perivascular sheath, which contains the nerves and the main blood vessels of the upper limb, local anaesthetic can spread up and down inside this sheath regardless of the point of needle insertion. Theoretically an identical block will be obtained if sufficient anaesthetic solution is injected. However, this may require an excessive amount of drug. Given in smaller amounts, each of the three approaches gives a somewhat different distribution of anaesthesia. The choice between the three therefore depends upon the individual patient and the type of surgery to be undertaken.

Because large doses of local anaesthetic, often exceeding the maximum recommended dose may be required, it is advisable to use drugs of low toxicity such as prilocaine or mepivacaine.

Interscalene brachial plexus block

Anatomy
The brachial plexus in the neck runs between the anterior and middle scalene muscles. The perivascular sheath containing the plexus can be reached at the level of the 6th cervical vertebra, i.e. the same level as the cricoid cartilage. This is some distance from either the subclavian artery or the dome of the pleura (Figs. 91:1a and b).

Patient position
Supine with upper limb at side. Head rotated a little away from the side to be blocked.

Landmarks
1. The groove between the anterior and middle scalene muscles. This is usually easily palpated behind the sternomastoid muscle, which is identified by asking the patient to raise his/her head. The muscle immediately behind the sternomastoid is the anterior scalene and by rolling the fingers backwards, the groove will be felt before reaching the middle scalene muscle.

2. Cricoid cartilage. This gives the level at which the needle should be inserted into the interscalene groove (Fig. 91:2).

Figs. 91:1 a and b.
1. First rib
2. Clavicle
3. Subclavian vein
4. Subclavian artery
5. Anterior scalene muscle
6. Middle scalene muscle
7. Transverse process of C6

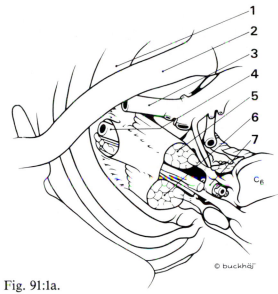

1
2
3
4
5
6
7

C₆

Fig. 91:1a.

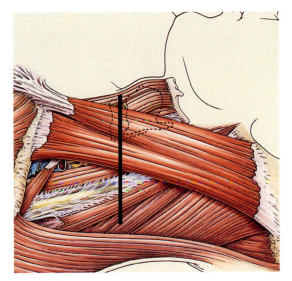

Fig. 91:2.

Fig. 91:1b.

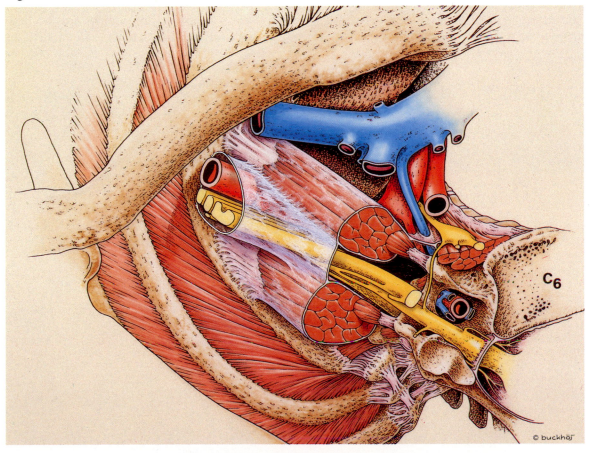

C₆

Needle insertion

A short needle (3-4 cm) may be used and is inserted perpendicular to the skin, i.e. medially but slightly downward and backward (Fig. 93:1). The index and middle finger of the non-dominant hand should be palpating the interscalene groove and preventing movement of the skin during needle insertion, which should be slightly closer to the middle than to the anterior scalene muscle. The needle is advanced **slowly** until a paraesthesia is elicited (Figs. 93:2 and 93:3), or a transverse spinous process is contacted. The paraesthesia must be felt **below the shoulder**, as those felt above the clavicle may be due to contact with the supraclavicular nerve, which is outside the perivascular sheath. If bone (the transverse process of the cervical vertebra) is contacted without paraesthesia it should be withdrawn slightly and "walked" laterally along the transverse process until a paraesthesia is elicited. The **downward** direction of the needle is important as it will prevent the spinal canal being entered with consequent inadvertent spinal or epidural block.

A nerve stimulator may be used with an appropriate insulated needle (see p. 28). Muscle twitching in the arm or hand (but **not** the shoulder girdle) indicates close proximity to the nerves of the plexus.

Injection

It is advisable to ask an assistant to make the injection using a flexible cannula so that neither the hand holding the needle nor the palpating hand need be moved during the injection (see "Immobile needle", p. 29). A very small amount (0.5 ml) should be injected first (after initial aspiration to eliminate the possibility of intravascular injection) and the patient questioned about any pain which would indicate a direct intraneural injection. If such pain occurs the needle should be withdrawn about 1 mm and the injection repeated. If no pain is experienced the main injection is given. The first 10 ml can be injected rapidly to elicit a dull ache in the neck, confirming the entrance of local anaesthetic into the perivascular sheath. The rest of the solution can be given more slowly, with several attempts to aspirate blood. No drug should be seen or felt to enter the subcutaneous tissues which would indicate too superficial an injection. Immediately after the injection the groove should be massaged both upwards and downwards.

Complete anaesthesia may take 30-40 min but signs of a developing block should occur within a few minutes. Tingling and a feeling of warmth in the limb are the first to appear. A sympathetic block with a warm hand and dilated veins compared to the unblocked side appears soon after. The first sign of motor block is seen in the shoulder.

Any deficiency in the anaesthesia can be made up with supplementary blocks at the wrist or elbow.

Drugs and dose

30-40 ml of 1.5% prilocaine or 0.375% bupivacaine, or their equivalent (see p. 20). Epinephrine 1:200.000 may be added for increased effect and longer duration. Carbonated solutions give more profound blocks than hydrochlorides.

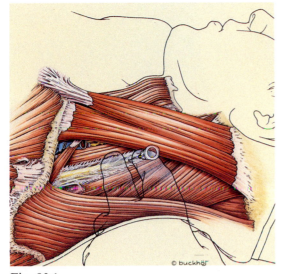

Fig. 93:1.

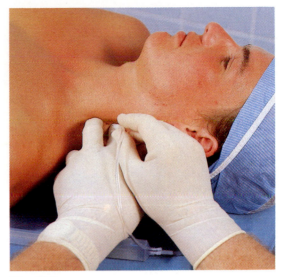

Fig. 93:2.

Fig. 93:3.

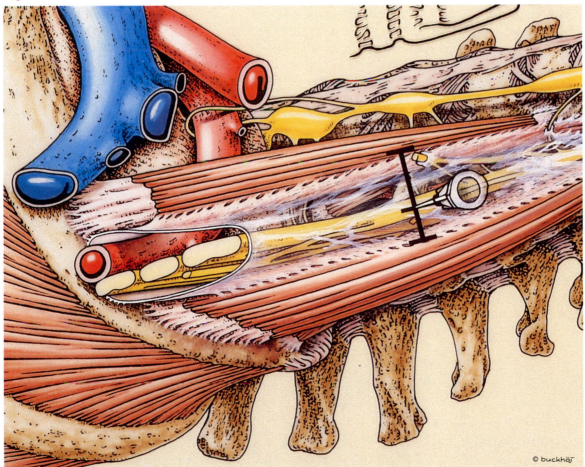

Complications

Spinal or epidural blockade
This can occur if the needle is directed cephalad instead of caudad, and enters an intervertebral foramen (Fig. 95:1). It may also occur in some patients with an exceptionally long dural cuff extending some distance from the intervertebral foramen (Fig. 95:2).

Epidural block will be diagnosed from the relatively slow onset of bilateral anaesthesia of the neck and thorax. Hypotension may occur and should be treated with a vasopressor, and/or IV fluids; otherwise no other therapy will be required.

Spinal anaesthesia will occur rapidly and may be associated with apnoea and unconsciousness. The respiration must be assisted or controlled and the blood pressure supported until the block wears off, which may take 1-2 h depending upon the dose and drug used (see p. 191).

Acute generalised toxicity (see p. 22)
Because a large volume and dose of drug is being used, toxicity may be a problem. Care must be taken to ensure that the recommended volume and concentration is used. If toxicity does occur, it will probably be seen 10-20 min after completing the injection. Inadvertent IV injection is unlikely, especially if frequent aspirations are made. Inadvertent intra-arterial injection, e.g. into the vertebral artery, will cause a rapid and severe reaction with convulsions after injecting only a few millilitres of solution, as the drug goes direct and undiluted to the brain. Again, arterial puncture should be easily recognised by aspiration.

Intraneural injection
Provided the initial small injection elicits the diagnosis, no permanent damage should ensue. Intraneural injection of larger amounts of drug can cause prolonged neuropathy.

very painful

Fig. 95:1.
1. *Stopped by bone*
2. *Puncture of the vertebral vessel*
3. *Needle in spinal canal*

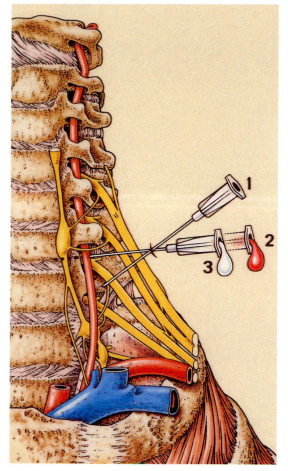

Fig. 95:1.

© buckhöj

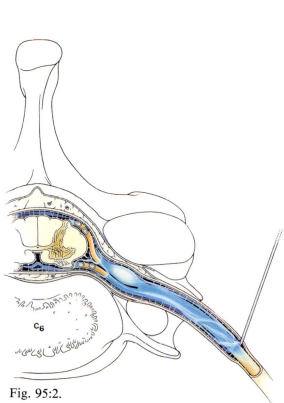

Fig. 95:2.

c₆

Supraclavicular brachial plexus block

There are several methods of supraclavicular brachial plexus block. The one described here is the subclavian perivascular block of Winnie which is much less likely to produce pneumothorax than other techniques.

Anatomy

As the brachial plexus passes between the clavicle and the first rib, it is joined by the subclavian artery, which runs deep to the anterior scalene muscle. The three trunks of the plexus are, as their names (superior, middle and inferior) imply, in a **vertical** plane lateral to the subclavian artery (Figs. 97:1a and b).

Patient position

Supine with arms at the side and head turned slightly away from the side to be injected. The arm on the injected side may be pulled downward to depress the clavicle and the shoulder, but the muscles should be relaxed.

Landmarks

1. Subclavian artery just above the junction of the medial and middle parts of the clavicle. Normally it can be identified by palpation of the arterial pulse (Figs. 97:2 and 97:3). In fat or muscular necks, it is often not possible to feel, but can be easily identified with an ultrasound probe (see p. 28).

2. The interscalene groove (see p. 90) posterior to the sternomastoid muscle.

Fig. 97:1.
1. First rib
2. Subclavian vein
3. Subclavian artery
4. Inferior trunk
5. Middle trunk
6. Superior trunk
7. Anterior scalene muscle
8. Middle scalene muscle
9. Transverse process of C6

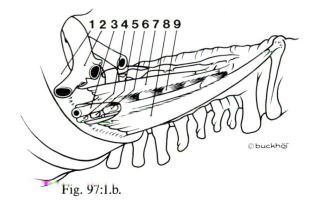

Fig. 97:1.a.

Fig. 97:1.b.

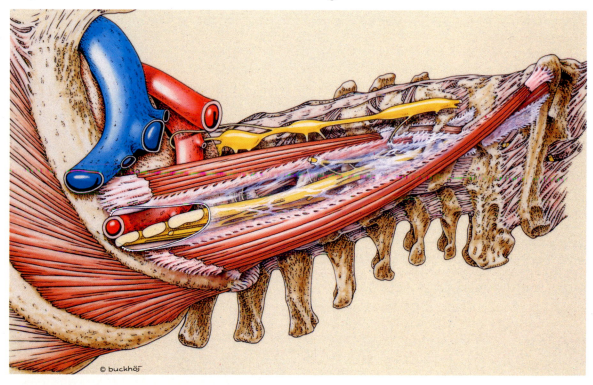

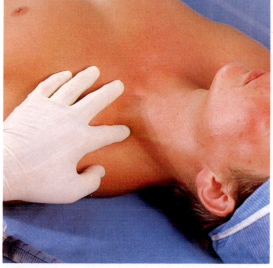

Fig. 97:2.

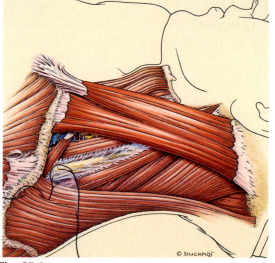

Fig. 97:3.

Needle insertion

The interscalene groove should be identified just above the clavicle by an index finger (the left for a left-sided block and the right for a right-sided block). The needle (4 cm, short bevelled) is inserted just above the palpating finger immediately lateral to the subclavian artery (Figs. 99:1 and 99:2). It is directed vertically downwards towards the patient's feet (Fig. 99:3). It should not proceed medially, laterally or posteriorly. It is advanced slowly until a paraesthesia, **felt below the shoulder**, is obtained. If no paraesthesia is obtained, the needle will eventually contact the first rib. It should be withdrawn and the process repeated as close as possible to the artery. As long as the needle does not point backwards and medially there is no danger of penetrating the pleura. Alternatively a nerve stimulator can be used (see p. 28) with an insulated needle, and muscular twitching in the arm or hand (**not** the shoulder girdle) indicates correct placement, and paraesthesia need not be elicited.

Injection

Once a paraesthesia is felt, or muscular twitching elicited with the nerve stimulator, **below** the shoulder, needle advancement is stopped and the syringe and plastic extension tube attached (see p. 29) by an assistant. 0.5 ml of local anaesthetic is injected quickly. If a sudden and severe pain is felt, the needle is intraneural and must be withdrawn 1-2 mm. If no such pain occurs, the main injection is given and it frequently causes a dull aching pain (''pressure paraesthesia'') confirming correct placement in the neurovascular sheath.

A sympathetic blockade causing warmth and dilated veins in the hand and arm occur within a few minutes. Motor weakness will appear in 5-10 min but it may take 20-40 min to produce full anaesthetic effect. Any deficiency in the anaesthesia can be made up with individual nerve blocks at the wrist or elbow.

Drugs and dose

30-50 ml of 1.5% lidocaine, 0.375% bupivacaine or their equivalent (see p. 20) with epinephrine 1:200.000. When larger volumes (40 ml or more) are used, the less toxic drugs prilocaine or mepivacaine are advised.
   Carbonated solutions give more profound blocks than hydrochlorides.

Complications

Arterial puncture
This indicates the needle is too anteromedial. Of itself it is not harmful, though a haematoma may occur. The needle must be withdrawn from the artery and moved more posterolateral, still keeping in the same strictly caudad direction.

Intraneural injection
Provided the initial small injection elicits the diagnosis, no permanent damage should ensue. Intraneural injection of larger amounts of drug can cause prolonged neuropathy.

Pneumothorax
Pneumothorax or accidental spinal/epidural block should not occur if the needle is correctly directed. If a large amount of air enters the pleural cavity, the classical signs and symptoms of pneumothorax will occur (Fig. 99:4). Otherwise an X-ray will be required to make the diagnosis.

Acute generalised toxicity
Acute generalised toxicity (see p. 22). Because a large volume and dose of drug is being used, toxicity may be a problem. Care must be taken to ensure the recommended volume and concentration are used. If it does occur, toxicity will probably be seen 10-20 min after completing the injection. Inadvertent IV injection is unlikely, especially if frequent aspirations are made.

Spinal/epidural block (see p. 94)
This may occur in patients with exceptionally long dural cuffs but is much less common than with interscalene block (see p. 95).

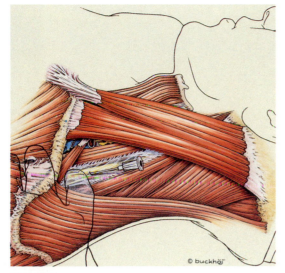

Fig. 99:1.

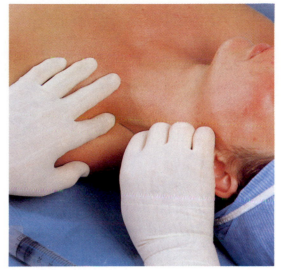

Fig. 99:2.

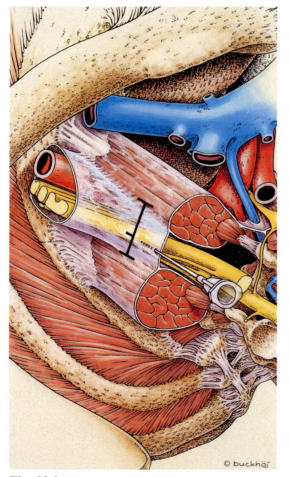

Fig. 99:3.

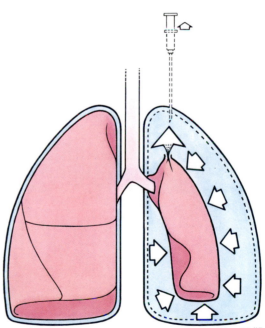

Fig. 99:4.

Axillary brachial plexus block

Axillary block is the most commonly used method of brachial plexus block, probably because it is not associated with pneumothorax. Unless large volumes are injected, it is less likely to anaesthetise the shoulder than the other methods.

Anatomy

After passing from the neck between the clavicle and first rib, the brachial plexus enters the upper limb via the axilla (Fig. 101:1). At this point the trunks of the plexus have each divided into an anterior and a posterior division which combine to form the three cords, lateral, medial and posterior. All the nerves are in close relationship to the axillary artery and lie within the perivascular sheath (Fig. 101:3). In the lower axilla, the trunks divide and form the four main terminal branches, the median, radial, ulnar and musculocutaneous nerves. The last mentioned quickly leaves the perivascular sheath through the coracobrachialis muscle (Fig. 101:2).

Patient position

The upper limb on the injected side should be abducted at the shoulder and flexed at right angles at the elbow so that the wrist is at the same level as the patient's head (Fig. 101:4). The hand should not be **under** the head, as this compresses the structures as they pass close to the coracoid process.

Landmarks

The axillary artery should be palpated and followed as high up into the axilla as possible. If the arterial pulsation is difficult to feel, ultrasound will accurately identify the artery (see p. 28).

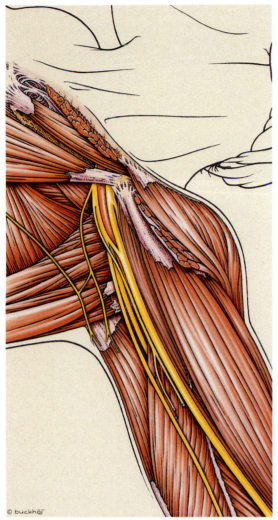

Fig. 101:1.

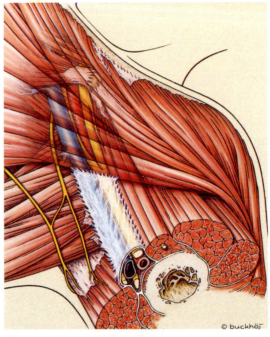

Fig. 101:2.

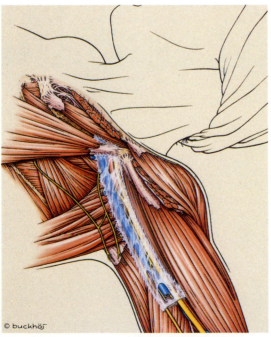

Fig. 101:3.

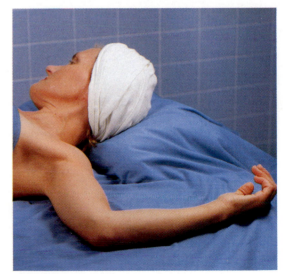

Fig. 101:4.

Needle insertion

A 4-cm short bevelled needle, attached to a plastic extension tube, is used. If a nerve stimulator is to be used, an insulated needle is preferred (see p. 28). The axillary artery is palpated continuously and the needle inserted just above the artery. It is directed towards the apex of the axilla, i.e. in almost the same plane as the neuromuscular bundle (Figs. 103:1 and 103:2). The needle is advanced slowly, keeping close to the artery until a paraesthesia is felt, or twitching of muscles in the arm or hand is seen with a nerve stimulator (see p. 28). Penetration of the neurovascular sheath is usually felt as a definite "give" as the needle is advanced. If the needle is then left untouched, it will be seen to move with each arterial beat, confirming its close relationship to the artery (Fig. 103:3).

If the needle enters the artery it may be withdrawn and realigned. Some authorities enter the artery on purpose, the needle being directed at right angles to the artery. When arterial blood is seen, the needle is advanced so as to exit the artery opposite its entry point and where it will be within the perivascular sheath (Fig. 103:4).

It should be possible to insert a catheter through the needle and into the perivascular sheath. There should be no obstruction to the forward movement of the catheter if the needle is correctly placed.

Injection

Using an assistant, the syringe is attached to the extension tube and if aspiration of blood is negative, 0.5 ml is injected. Acute severe pain following this indicates an intraneural injection and the needle must be withdrawn 1-2 mm. If no pain occurs, the main injection should be given. Little or no resistance to the injection should be encountered. It may cause a dull ache due to pressure within the perivascular sheath. To encourage the local anaesthetic solution to travel upwards in the sheath and not downwards, the palpating finger is pressed firmly on the artery distal to the needle during and after the injection.

A sympathetic blockade causing warmth and dilated veins in the hand and arm occurs within a few minutes. Motor weakness will appear in 5-10 min but it may take 20-40 min to produce the full effect. Any deficiency in the anaesthesia can be made up with individual nerve blocks at the wrist or elbow.

Drugs and dose

30-40 ml of 1.5% lidocaine or 0.375% bupivacaine or their equivalent (see p. 20) with epinephrine 1:200.000. With the larger volumes, prilocaine or mepivacaine are to be preferred on account of their lower toxicity.

Carbonated solutions give more profound blocks than hydrochlorides.

Complications

Acute generalised toxicity

Acute generalised toxicity (see p. 22). Because a large volume and dose of drug is being used, toxicity may be a problem. Care must be taken to ensure the recommended volume and concentration are used. If it does occur, toxicity will probably be seen 10-20 min after completing the injection. Inadvertent IV injection is unlikely, especially if frequent aspirations are made, but if it occurs overt toxicity will be seen within a few minutes.

Intraneural injection

Provided the initial small injection elicits the diagnosis, no permanent damage should ensue. Intraneural injection of larger amounts of drug can cause prolonged neuropathy.

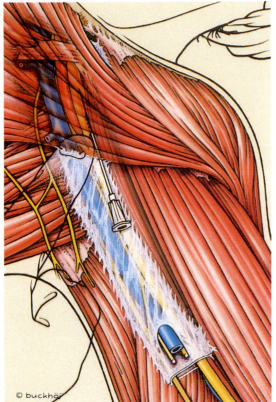

Fig. 103:1.
Fig. 103:3.

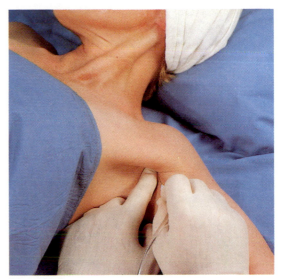

Fig. 103:2.
Fig. 103:4.

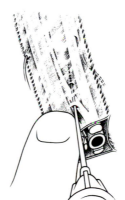
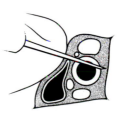

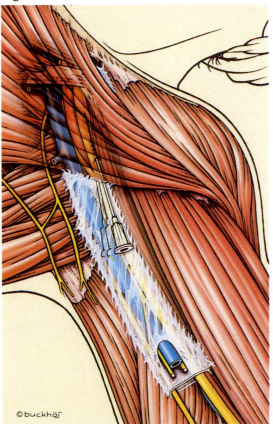

Supplementary blocks with brachial plexus block

Brachial plexus block occasionally fails to produce complete analgesia of the upper limb. After 20-30 min it will become obvious that an individual nerve in the plexus has not been blocked. Supplementary blocks can easily be done lower down the arm in such an eventuality.

Inadequate anaesthesia in the ulnar nerve distribution is sometimes seen with interscalene block and this will require a further block of the ulnar nerve at the elbow (see p. 106). The median and radial nerves may also be blocked at the elbow (see p. 108 and p. 110).

In addition, blockade of the brachial plexus alone within the perivascular sheath still leaves the skin of the inner side of the upper arm unanaesthetised. This area is supplied by:

1. The intercostobrachial nerve (which is the lateral cutaneous branch of the second intercostal nerve and therefore derives from T2)

2. The medial brachial cutaneous nerve, which leaves the perivascular sheath high up in the axilla

If it is considered necessary to anaesthetise this area, it can be done simply by a subcutaneous injection in the axilla. Because a tourniquet is often placed on this part of the upper arm, the discomfort of the tourniquet may be relieved by the additional injection. However, tourniquet pain is caused mostly by muscle ischaemia and with a good brachial plexus block, tourniquet pain is seldom a problem.

Intercostobrachial nerve block

Anatomy
The intercostobrachial and the medial brachial cutaneous nerves cross the axilla and pierce the deep fascia to reach the skin of the medial side of the upper arm (Fig. 105:1).

Patient position
Supine. Arm at right angle to the trunk, with the elbow also at right angle (Fig. 105:2).

Landmarks
The axillary artery should be palpated.

Needle insertion
The needle is inserted over the axillary artery and advanced subcutaneously in a caudal direction, at right angles to the artery, for a distance of 3-4 cm (Fig. 105:2 and 3). Following an axillary block, it is not necessary to totally withdraw the needle, which, just below its insertion point, is redirected at right angles.

Drugs and dose
3-5 ml of local anaesthetic is injected subcutaneously while withdrawing the needle.

Suggested further reading
Selander, D., Edshage, S. & Wolff, T. (1979) Paresthesia or no paresthesia? Nerve Resions after axillary blocks. Acta Anaesth. Scand. 23, 27.
Winnie, A.P. (1983) Plexus Anesthesia I. Schultz, Copenhagen.

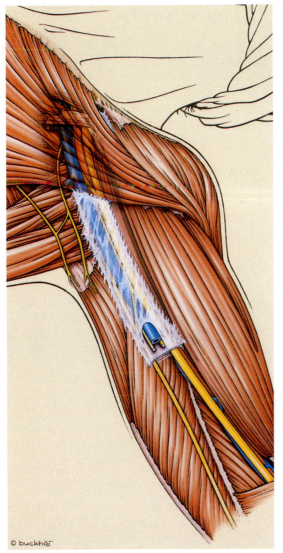

© buckhöj

Fig. 105:1.

Fig. 105:2.

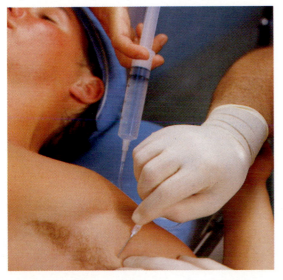

Fig. 105:3.

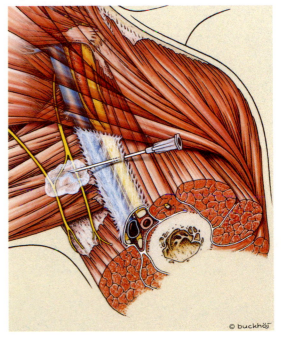

© buckhöj

Nerve blocks at the elbow

Brachial plexus block sometimes produces less than ideal anaesthesia in the lower arm and hand. This may be due to:

1. Inadequate dosage

2. Atypical spread of the local anaesthetic within the perivascular sheath

3. Inadequate penetration of the large nerves of the plexus, it being the inside or "core" fibres which innervate the lower arm and hand

While waiting for a brachial plexus block to become fully effective it may be possible to detect the slow and inadequate development of anaesthesia in the distribution of one of the larger nerves. The ulnar nerve, for example, may not always be blocked by an interscalene injection. It is not difficult in such cases to block any of the three major nerves at the elbow to reinforce a brachial plexus block.

Blockade of the ulnar, median and radial nerves at the elbow is relatively easy and will anaesthetise the lower forearm and hand, including the deep structures such as the bones, joints, ligaments and tendons (Figs. 107:1, 107:2, 109:1, 109:2, 111:1 and 111:2).

Ulnar nerve block

Anatomy
The ulnar nerve is easily palpable (the "funny bone") behind the medial epicondyle of the humerus and lateral to the olecranon. It enters the forearm between the two heads of flexor carpi ulnaris.

Patient position
Elbow flexed at right angles.

Landmarks
1. Medial epicondyle of humerus
2. Olecranon
3. Ulnar nerve itself can usually be felt.

Needle insertion
Insert needle through skin and advance towards (but not pierce) the nerve which is fixed by the other hand. A paraesthesia may be elicited or a nerve stimulator can be used (Figs. 107:3 and 107:4).

After aspiration inject 0.5 ml initially. If sudden severe pain is produced the needle is intraneural and should be withdrawn 1-2 mm. If there is no such pain, the main injection can proceed.

Drugs and dose
5 ml of 1% lidocaine or 0.25% bupivacaine or their equivalent (see p. 20). Epinephrine 1:200.000 can be added.

Fig. 107:1.
1. Flexor carpi ulnaris muscle — C8-T1
2. Flexor digitorum profundus muscle — C8-T1
3. Abductor digiti minimi muscle — C8-T1
4. Flexor digiti minimi brevis muscle — C8-T1
5. Opponens digiti minimi muscle — C8-T1
6. Lumbrical muscle — C6-C8
7. Flexor pollicis brevis muscle — C6-T1
8. Adductor pollicis muscle — C8-T1
9. Palmar interossei muscles — C8-T1
10. Dorsal interossei muscles — C8-T1

Fig. 107:4. Courtesy of Astra.

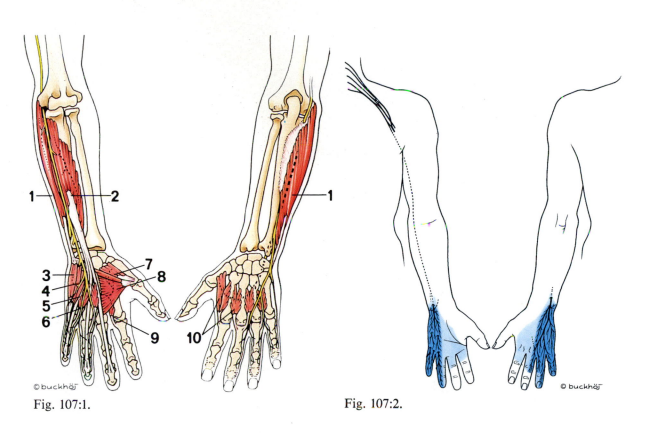

1
2
3
4
5
6
7
8
9
10

Fig. 107:1.

Fig. 107:2.

Fig. 107:3.

Fig. 107:4.

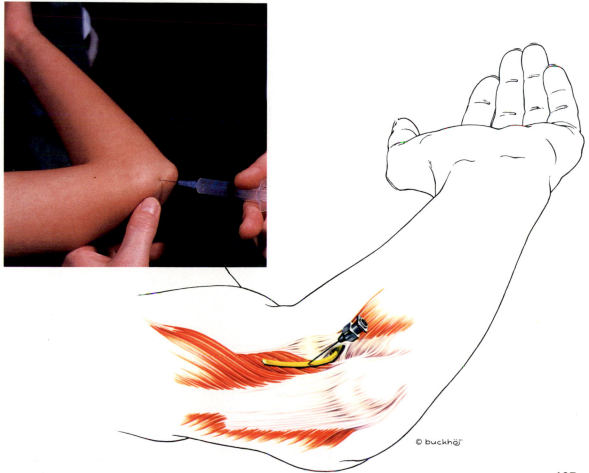

Median nerve block

Anatomy
At the elbow, the median nerve lies medial to the brachial artery between the bicipital aponeurosis and the brachialis muscle. It enters the forearm between the two heads of pronator teres (Fig. 109:4).

Patient position
Elbow extended.

Landmarks
1. Medial and lateral epicondyles of humerus
2. Brachial artery

Needle insertion
Palpate the brachial artery 1-2 cm above the line joining the two epicondyles. Insert the needle lateral to the artery passing through the deep fascia (Figs. 109:3 and 109:4). Paraesthesia may be obtained or a nerve stimulator used.

After aspiration inject 0.5 ml initially. If sudden severe pain is produced the needle is intraneural and should be withdrawn 1-2 mm. If there is no such pain, the main injection can proceed.

Drugs and dose
5 ml of 1% lidocaine or 0.25% bupivacaine or their equivalent (see p. 20). Epinephrine 1:200.000 can be added.

Fig. 109:2.

1. Flexor digitorum profundus muscle	C8-T1
2. Flexor pollicis longus muscle	C8-T1
3. Pronator quadratus muscle	C8-T1
4. Opponens pollicis muscle	C6-C7
5. Lumbrical muscles	C6-C8
6. Flexor digitorum superficialis muscle	C8-T1
7. Abductor pollicis brevis muscle	C6-C7
8. Flexor pollicis brevis muscle	C6-T1
9. Pronator teres muscle	C6-C7
10. Palmaris longus muscle	C6-C7
11. Flexor carpi radialis muscle	C6-C7

Fig. 109:4. Courtesy of Astra.
1. Median nerve
2. Lateral cutaneous nerve of the forearm
3. Radial nerve
4. Brachial artery
5. Tendon of biceps muscle
6. Brachioradialis muscle

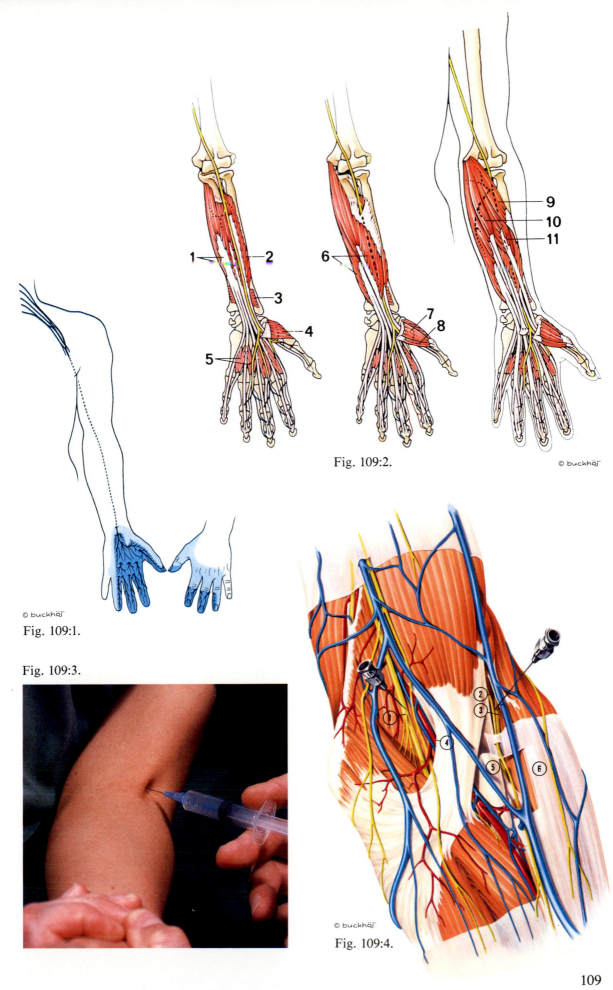

Fig. 109:1.

Fig. 109:2.

© buckhöj

Fig. 109:3.

Fig. 109:4.

© buckhöj

109

Radial nerve block

Anatomy
At the level of the lateral epicondyle of the humerus, the radial nerve lies 1 cm lateral to the biceps tendon, and medial to the brachioradialis muscle. Because the nerve is in close relationship to the musculo-cutaneous nerve, both nerves will usually be blocked (Fig. 111:3).

Patient position
Elbow extended.

Landmarks
1. Lateral epicondyle
2. Biceps tendon
3. Brachioradialis muscle

Needle insertion
Palpate the cleft between the biceps tendon and the brachioradialis muscle and insert the needle into the cleft until a paraesthesia is elicited or it contacts the lateral epicondyle (Fig. 111:3 and 4). If no paraesthesia is obtained, redirect and advance towards the condyle in a more lateral direction. When a paraesthesia is elicited, inject after aspiration. A nerve stimulator may be used instead of eliciting paraesthesia.

Drugs and dose
5 ml of 1% lidocaine, or 0.25% bupivacaine or their equivalent (see p. 20). Epinephrine 1:200.000 may be added.

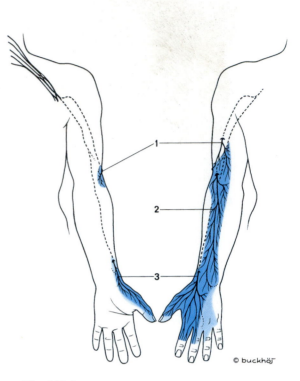

Fig. 110:1

Fig. 110:1.
1. Dorsal brachial cutaneous nerve	C5-C6
2. Dorsal antebrachial cutaneous nerve	C5-C8
3. Cutaneouos distribution	C6-C8

Figs. 111:1 and 111:2
1. Triceps brachii muscle	C7-C8
2. Supinator muscle	C6
3. Extensor carpi radialis brevis muscle	C6-C7
4. Abductor pollicis longus muscle	C6-C7
5. Anconeus muscle	C7-C8
6. Extensor pollicis longus muscle	C6-C8
7. Extensor indicis muscle	C6-C8
8. Extensor pollicis brevis muscle	C6-C7
9. Brachioradialis muscle	C5-C6
10. Extensor carpi radialis longus muscle	C6-C7
11. Extensor digitorum muscle	C6-C8
12. Extensor carpi ulnaris muscle	C6-C8
13. Extensor digiti minimi muscle	C6-C8

Fig. 111:3. Courtesy of Astra.
1. Median nerve
2. Lateral cutaneous nerve of the forearm
3. Radial nerve
4. Brachial artery
5. Tendon of biceps muscle
6. Brachioradialis muscle

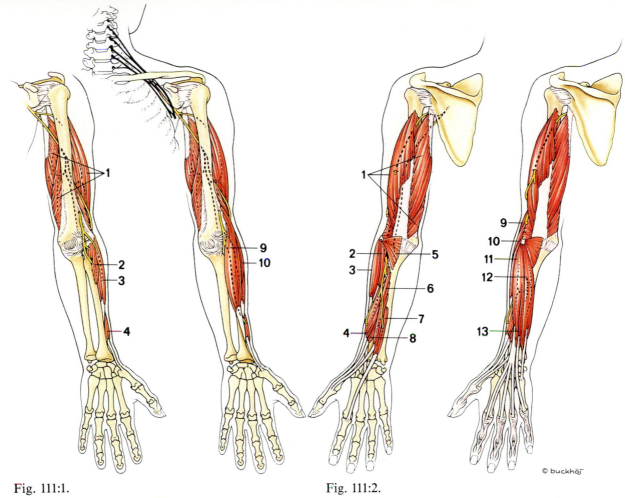

Fig. 111:1.

Fig. 111:2.

© buckhöj

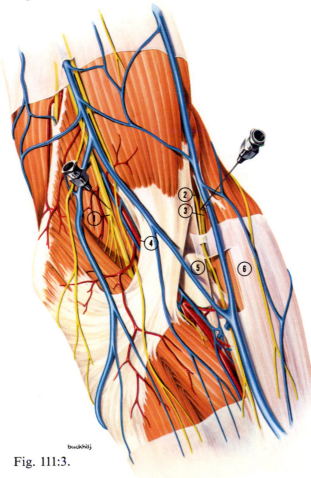

Fig. 111:3.

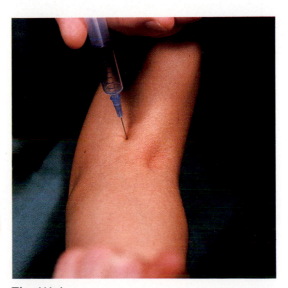

Fig. 111:4.

Nerve blocks at the wrist

The terminal branches of the ulnar, median and radial nerves are all easily blocked at the wrist and can be used either for surgery of the hand or to reinforce a brachial plexus block. The ulnar and median nerves are still beneath the deep fascia at the wrist but are closely related to easily identified tendons. They supply the deep structures of the hand anteriorly (i.e. the bones, joints and muscles) as well as the skin (Fig. 113:1). The radial nerve, however, is in the superficial fascia and consequently only innervates skin. The deep structures of the hand posteriorly are supplied by the superior interosseous nerve, which leaves the radial nerve high up in the forearm. Nerve blocks at the wrist should therefore only be used for operations on the skin, or for postoperative pain relief. Because of the small size of the nerves it is not necessary or desirable to elicit paraesthesia.

Median nerve

This lies between the palmaris longus tendon and the tendon of flexor carpi radialis. The needle is inserted vertical to the skin and close to the lateral border of palmaris longus, to pierce the deep fascia (Figs. 113:2 and 113:3).

Drugs and dose
2-3 ml of 1% lidocaine or its equivalent (see p. 20) will suffice.

Ulnar nerve

This lies just lateral to (i.e. on the radial side of) the flexor carpi ulnaris tendon at the level of the styloid process of the ulnar bone. The needle is inserted vertical to the skin just lateral to the tendon, to pierce the deep fascia. (Figs. 113:2 and 113:3).

Drugs and dose
Inject 2-3 ml of 1% lidocaine or its equivalent (see p. 20).

Radial nerve

This lies in the superficial fascia at the wrist, where it will have divided into its terminal branches. These can all be blocked by subcutaneous infiltration between the radial artery anteriorly and the extensor carpi radialis tendon posteriorly. The needle may be inserted at the middle of this band of infiltration directed first one way and then the other (Fig. 113:4).

Drugs and dose
5 ml of 0.5-1% lidocaine or its equivalent (see p. 20) will suffice.

Fig. 113:2.
1. Median nerve
2. Tendon of the flexor carpi radialis muscle
3. Tendon of palmaris longus muscle
4. Ulnar artery
5. Ulnar nerve
6. Tendon of the flexor carpi ulnaris muscle

Figs. 113:1-4. Courtesy of Astra.

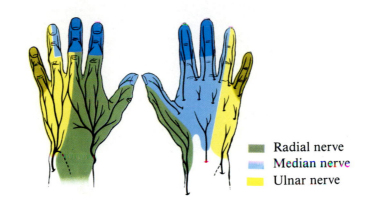

■	Radial nerve
■	Median nerve
■	Ulnar nerve

Fig. 113:1.

© buckhöj

Fig. 113:2.

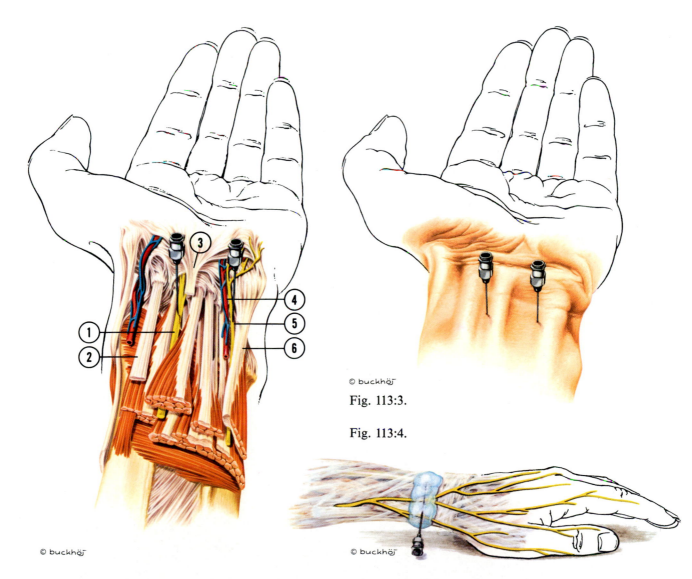

© buckhöj

© buckhöj

Fig. 113:3.

Fig. 113:4.

113

Digital nerve block of the finger

This is a simple and effective way of anaesthetising a finger.

Anatomy

Two digital nerves run on each side of each finger, a palmar and a dorsal branch (Figs. 114:1 and 115:1).

Needle insertion

The easiest method is to insert a needle at the base of the digit to contact the proximal phalanx at its lateral point (Fig. 115:2). Withdraw the needle fractionally and deposit 0.5 ml of local anaesthetic. Redirect the needle towards the dorsal part of the digit (Fig. 115:3) and inject a further 1 ml as the needle is slowly withdrawn. Repeating this on the palmar aspect of the digit (Fig. 115:4) will leave a semicircle of local anaesthetic. When repeated on the other side of the digit a complete ring of the injected drug will surround the base of the finger.

Alternatively the injection can be made proximal to the base of the digit to block the nerves as they run between the metacarpal bones. The needle is inserted 2 cm proximal to the web of the digit until it is within the space between the adjacent bones (Fig. 115:5). By palpating the space as the injection is made, the filling of the space will be felt. An intercarpal injection anaesthetises the adjacent sides of two digits and therefore to complete the anaesthesia of a whole digit the adjacent space must also be injected.

Drugs and dose

4 ml of lidocaine 1% or its equivalent. Epinephrine is not recommended in digital blocks.

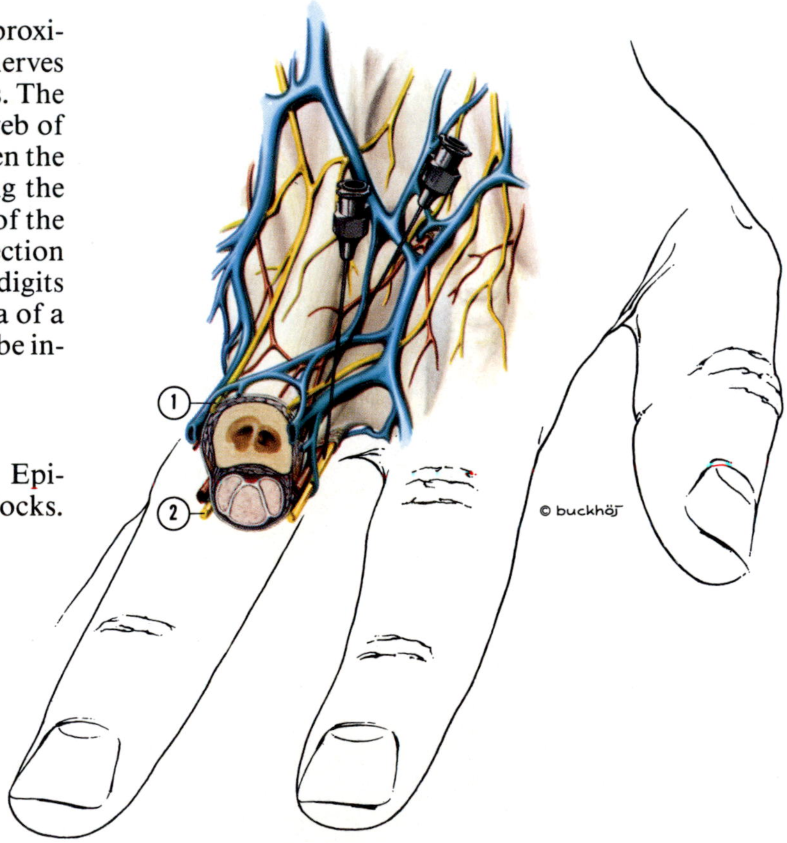

Fig. 114:1. Courtesy of Astra.
1. Dorsal digital nerve
2. Palmar digital nerve

Fig. 115:1.
1. Dorsal digital nerve

114

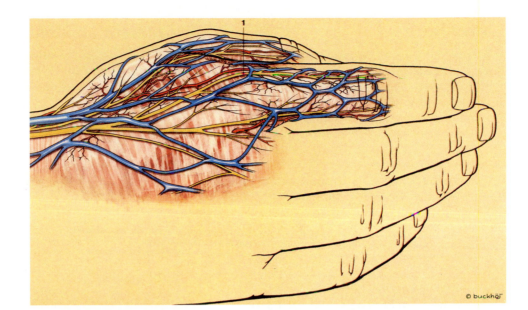

Fig. 115:1.

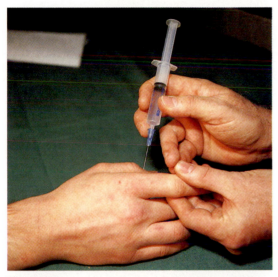

Fig. 115:2.

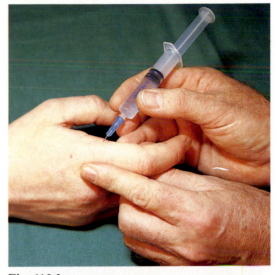

Fig. 115:3.

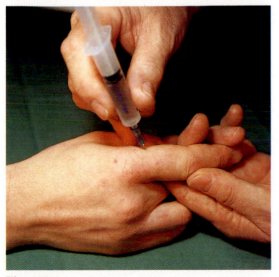

Fig. 115:4.

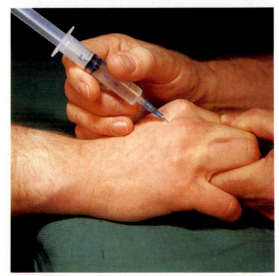

Fig. 115:5.

Lower limb

The lower limb can be rendered anaesthetic simply and effectively by spinal or epidural block. However, these techniques involve some degree of sympathetic blockade and there may be patients in whom this should be avoided. As with the upper limb, the nerves to the lower limb can be blocked at any part of their course from the spine to the periphery. The three main nerves are the sciatic, the femoral and the obturator nerves. The lateral cutaneous nerve of thigh is much smaller and supplies skin only. They all derive from the lumbar and sacral plexuses. The lumbar plexus (L2, 3, 4) gives rise to the femoral and obturator nerves and also to the lateral cutaneous nerve of the thigh. The lumbar plexus lies in the posterior part of the psoas muscle. The sacral plexus (L4, 5, S1, 2, 3 and 4) gives rise to the sciatic nerve. The sciatic nerve leaves the pelvis through the greater sciatic foramen and enters the back of the thigh between the greater trochanter of the femur and the tuberosity of the ischium. It divides, in the lower third of the posterior thigh, into its two main terminal branches, the tibial and common peroneal nerves.

The cutaneous distribution of the three largest nerves is shown in Fig. 117:2. All three nerves supply both the hip and the knee joints and to obtain complete anaesthesia of the lower limb it is necessary to block all three. A femoral nerve block by itself is effective in relieving the pain of a fractured shaft of femur, but not of the femoral neck. Block of the lateral cutaneous nerve of thigh alone allows skin grafts to be taken from the lateral thigh.

Sciatic nerve block

The sciatic nerve is the biggest nerve in the body but it lies deep in the posterior thigh. There are three main approaches to the nerve, anterior with the patient lying supine, posterior with the patient in the lateral position and posterior with the patient supine and the hip and knee joint flexed to right angles as in the lithotomy position (Raj approach). The choice will depend upon the ability to turn the patient appropriately without discomfort, e.g. for patients with fractured bones, the anterior approach is best. Whichever method is used, a nerve stimulator technique is strongly advised.

Anterior sciatic approach

This is particularly suitable for patients lying supine who cannot be turned laterally or have their hip and knee joints flexed, e.g. those with fractures.

Anatomy
While the sciatic nerve for much of its course lies behind the femur, it is medial to the bone at the level of the lesser trochanter and is therefore accessible to a needle inserted anteriorly.

Patient position
Supine.

Landmarks
1. Anterior superior iliac spine
2. Pubic tubercle
3. Greater trochanter

Draw a line from the anterior superior iliac spine to the pubic tubercle along the inguinal ligament, and a parallel line from the greater trochanter across the upper thigh. Connect the two parallel lines with a line at right angles to both from the junction of the medial and middle thirds of the upper line. The point where the connecting line joins the lower line marks the position of the lesser trochanter (Fig. 117:3).

Needle insertion
The usual description of the anterior approach advises needle insertion directly over the point marking the lesser trochanter. However, long needles bend easily, and after contacting the femoral shaft it is not easy to redirect towards the sciatic nerve. A more medial insertion is therefore advisable. A long (12-15 cm) needle is inserted perpendicularly downwards through the skin **1 cm medial** to the point which marks the position of the lesser trochanter (Fig. 117:1).

Push the needle in a vertical direction (with the patient supine) and slightly laterally to contact the lesser trochanter or the shaft of the femur (Fig. 117:1 and 4). Withdraw almost to the skin and realign until the needle passes medially to the femur. The sciatic nerve will be found about 5 cm behind the femur. Using a nerve stimulator observe the foot for movement during stimulation. The needle point is moved to the optimal position (see p. 28).

Figs. 117:1. Courtesy of Astra.

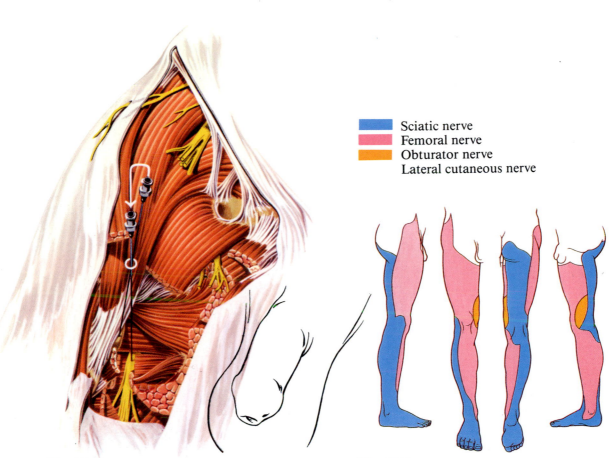

Fig. 117:1.

© buckhöj

Fig. 117:2.

© buckhöj

Fig. 117:3.

Fig. 117:4.

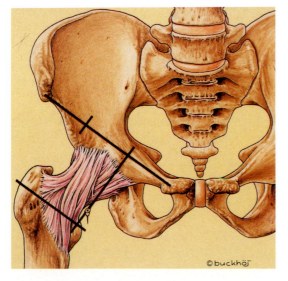

© buckhöj

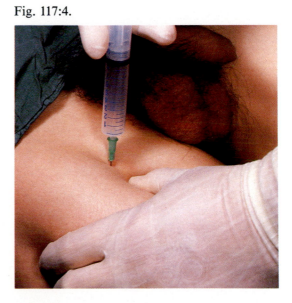

Drugs and dose

15-20 ml of 1.5% lidocaine or 0.375% bupivacaine (or their equivalent, see p. 20). Epinephrine 1:200.000 may be added. If this nerve block is being combined with a femoral 3 in 1 block (see p. 122), then quite large amounts of local anaesthetic may need to be injected. In such cases prilocaine 1.5% is the drug of choice due to its low toxicity. As the two injections will be seperated by an interval of several minutes, the danger of toxicity will be considerably reduced.

Complications

1. Acute toxicity (see p. 22).
2. Intraneural injection with neuropathy (see p. 26).

Posterior approach

Anatomy

The sciatic nerve leaves the pelvis through the greater sciatic foramen and may be blocked just inferior to this, as it passes below the piriformis muscle.

Patient position

Lateral with side to be injected uppermost. The thigh and knee are flexed at right angles so that the limb lies in front of the dependent limb.

Landmarks

1. Posterior superior iliac spine
2. Greater trochanter

Join these with a line and draw a second line at right angles from its midpoint (Fig. 119:2).

Needle insertion

The needle should be inserted at a point 4 cm down the second line, through the gluteus maximus (Fig. 119:1 and 2). It is advanced slowly until the nerve stimulator causes movement of the foot, usually about 7-8 cm from the skin. The needle point is moved to the optimal position (see p. 28).

Drugs and dose

15-20 ml of 1.5% lidocaine or 0.375% bupivacaine (or their equivalent, see p. 20). Epinephrine 1:200.000 may be added. If this nerve block is being combined with a femoral 3 in 1 block, then quite large amounts of local anaesthetic may need to be injected. In such cases prilocaine 1.5% is the drug of choice due to its low toxicity. As the two injections will be separated by an interval of several minutes, the danger of toxicity will be considerably reduced.

Complications

1. Acute toxicity (see p. 22)
2. Intraneural injection with neuropathy (see p. 26)

Fig. 119:1.
1. Posterior superior iliac spine
2. Greater trochanter

Figs. 119:2 and 3. Courtesy of Astra.

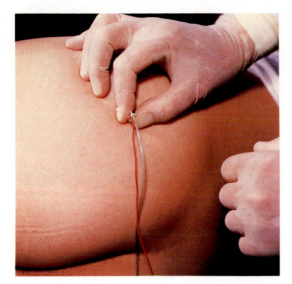

Fig. 119:1.

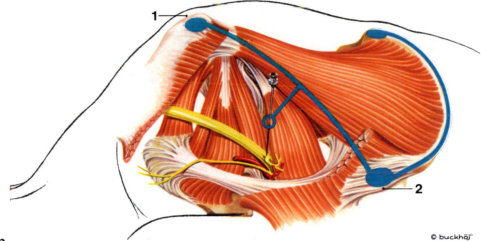

Fig. 119:2.

© buckhöj

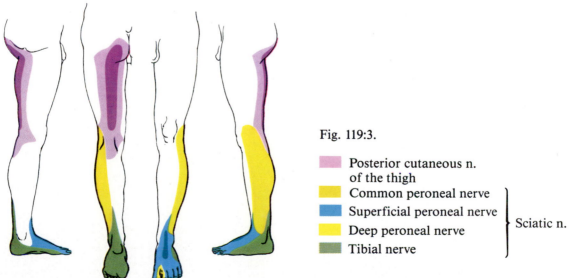

Fig. 119:3.

Posterior cutaneous n.
of the thigh

Common peroneal nerve

Superficial peroneal nerve

Deep peroneal nerve

Tibial nerve

} Sciatic n.

Posterior approach, Raj technique

Anatomy
In this approach the patient remains supine, but the lower limb is raised into the lithotomy position. In this position the sciatic nerve is stretched and therefore more firmly fixed as it passes between the greater trochanter and the ischial tuberosity. The nerve is thus blocked a little lower than in the classical posterior approach.

Patient position
Supine with the lower limb in the lithotomy position (hip and knee flexed to right angles). The limb may be held by an assistant (Fig. 121:1).

Landmarks
1. Greater trochanter
2. Ischial tuberosity

Needle insertion
The needle is inserted at right angles to the skin at the midpoint between the greater trochanter and the ischial tuberosity (Fig. 121:2). It is advanced until the nerve stimulator causes movement of the foot, and the needle point is in the optimal position (see p. 28).

Drugs and dose
15-20 ml of 1.5% lidocaine or 0.375% bupivacaine (or their equivalent, see p. 20). Epinephrine 1:200.000 may be added. If this nerve block is being combined with a femoral 3 in 1 block, then quite large amounts of local anaesthetic may need to be injected. In such cases prilocaine 1.5% is the drug of choice due to its low toxicity. As the two injections will be separated by an interval of several minutes, the danger of toxicity will be considerably reduced.

Complications
1. Acute toxicity (see p. 22)
2. Intraneural injection with neuropathy (see p. 26)

Fig. 121:3. Courtesy of Astra.

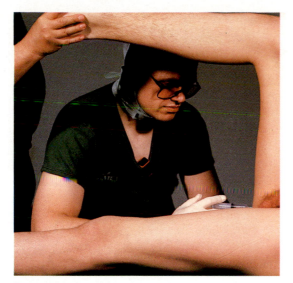

Fig. 121:1.

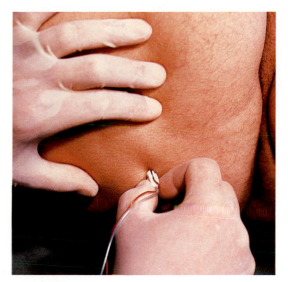

Fig. 121:2.

Fig. 121:3.

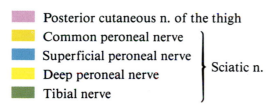

Posterior cutaneous n. of the thigh
Common peroneal nerve
Superficial peroneal nerve   } Sciatic n.
Deep peroneal nerve
Tibial nerve

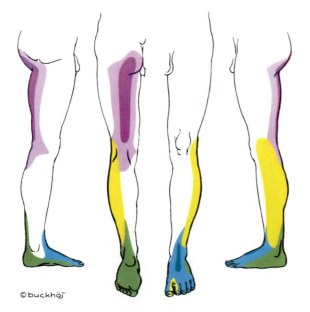

©buckhöj

Femoral, obturator and lateral cutaneous nerve block

Although these nerves may be blocked separately, it is now common practice to use the "3 in 1" block which will block the lumbar plexus including the femoral, obturator and lateral cutaneous nerve of thigh.

3 in 1 lumbar plexus block

This block anaesthetises the femoral, obturator and lateral cutaneous nerve of the thigh. When combined with a sciatic block, the entire lower limb is affected.

Anatomy

The lumbar plexus lies in the posterior part of the psoas muscle. The quadratus lumborum and iliacus muscles lie posteriorly. Like the brachial plexus, the lumbar plexus is enclosed within a sheath of connective tissue which can be entered at the level of the inguinal ligament where the femoral nerve enters the thigh (Fig. 123:1).

Local anaesthetic injected at this point will spread cephalad between the iliacus and psoas muscles, blocking all the branches of the lumbar plexus.

Patient position
Supine.

Landmarks
1. Inguinal ligament
2. Femoral artery

Needle insertion

The needle is inserted just below the inguinal ligament, 1-1.5 cm lateral to the femoral artery (Fig. 123:2). The needle is directed cephalad at about 60° from the skin, and advanced slowly until either a paraesthesia is elicited or a nerve stimulator causes movement of the patella.

Drugs and dose

25-30 ml of 1.5% lidocaine or 0.375% bupivacaine, or their equivalent (see p. 20). Epinephrine 1:200.000 can be added. If combined with sciatic nerve block, prilocaine 1-5% or mepivacaine 1.5% are recommended because of their lower toxicity. As the two injections will be seperated by an interval of several minutes, the danger of toxicity will be considerably reduced.

Complications
1. Acute toxicity (see p. 22)
2. Neuropathy due to intraneural injection (see p. 25)

Femoral nerve block

This is a particularly good block for patients with a fracture of the shaft of the femur as it allows painless reduction of the fracture and the application of the traction.

The technique is exactly the same as for the 3 in 1 block but less drug, 10-15 ml, is used.

Fig. 123:1.
1. Lateral cutaneous n. of the thigh
2. Femoral nerve

Fig. 123:1 and 3. Courtesy of Astra

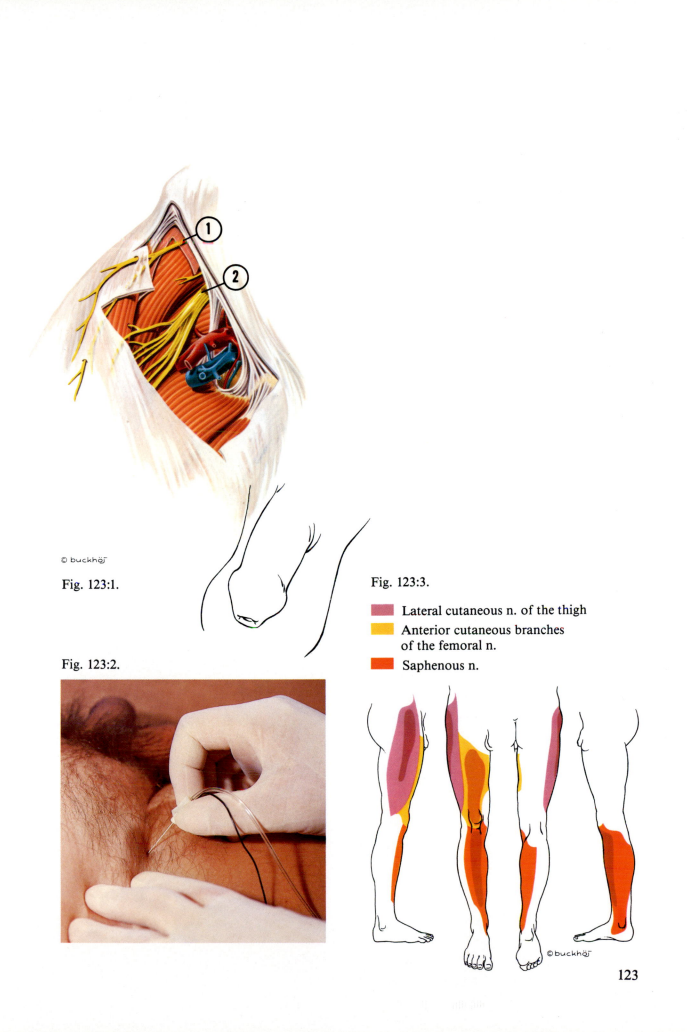

© buckhöj

Fig. 123:1.

Fig. 123:2.

Fig. 123:3.

Lateral cutaneous n. of the thigh

Anterior cutaneous branches of the femoral n.

Saphenous n.

© buckhöj

Obturator nerve block

Anatomy

The obturator nerve leaves the lumbar plexus through the psoas muscle, to reach the medial side of the muscle behind the common iliac vessels (Fig. 125:3). It runs downwards and forwards to reach the obturator foramen, entering the thigh through the upper part of the foramen just below the superior pubic ramus. It ends there by dividing into an anterior and a posterior branch (Fig. 125:4). The former supplies the anterior adductor muscles at the hip joint, before ending superficially in the skin on the medial aspect of the upper thigh. The posterior branch supplies the deep adductor muscles and sends an articular branch to the knee joint.

Patient position

Supine with the thigh partially abducted and the knee partially flexed.

Landmarks

Pubic tubercle

Needle insertion

The needle is inserted 1-2 cm lateral and inferior to the pubic tubercle, over the adductor longus tendon, which can be felt with the thigh abducted (Fig. 125:1). It is directed upwards, backwards and laterally to contact the pubic ramus. It is then redirected so as to pass just below the inferior border of the pubic ramus and into the obturator foramen (Fig. 125:2). If a nerve stimulator is used the adductor muscles will be seen to twitch.

Drugs and dose

10 ml of 1% lidocaine or 0.25% bupivacaine, or their equivalent (see p. 20). Epinephrine 1:200.000 can be added. If combined with sciatic and femoral block then prilocaine 1% should be used on account of its lower toxicity.

Fig. 125:4. Obturator nerve
1. *Anterior branch*
2. *Posterior branch*
3. *Pectineus muscle*
4. *Adductor brevis muscle*
5. *Adductor longus muscle*
6. *Gracilis muscle*
7. *Cutaneous branch*
8. *Branch to the hip joint*
9. *Adductor magnus muscle*
10. *Branch to the knee joint*

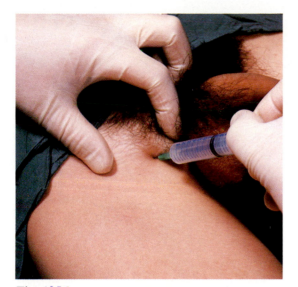

Fig. 125:1.

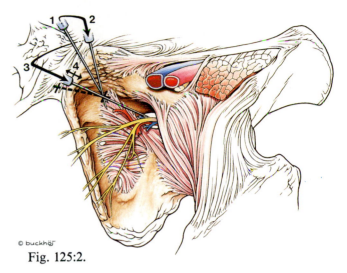

Fig. 125:2.

Fig. 125:3.

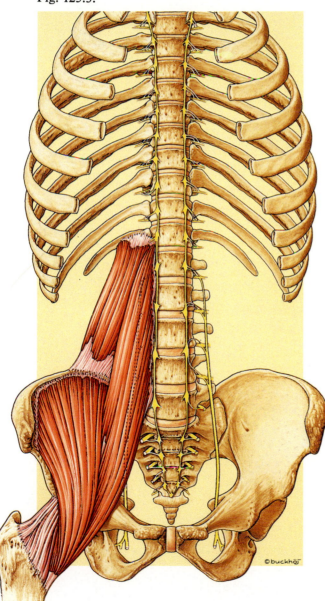

Fig. 125:4.

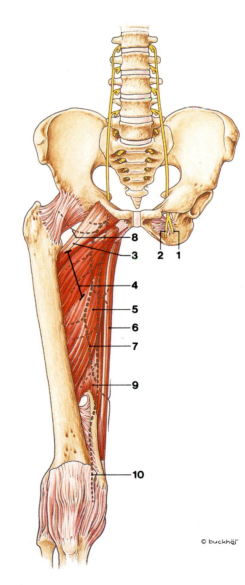

Lateral cutaneous nerve of thigh block

Anatomy

The lateral cutaneous nerve of thigh leaves the lumbar plexus and runs lateral to the psoas muscle on iliacus. It passes under the inguinal ligament 1 cm medial to the anterior superior iliac spine, lying beneath the fascia lata (Fig. 127:1). It supplies the skin on the lateral side of the thigh (Fig. 127:3).

Patient position

Supine.

Landmarks

Anterior superior iliac spine

Needle insertion

The needle is inserted 2 cm medial and inferior to the anterior superior iliac spine (Fig. 127:2). The needle is directed cephalad to pierce the fascia lata and contact the iliac crest. Inject 3-5 ml of local anaesthetic between the crest and the fascia lata. Repeat the injection twice, moving the needle more medially on each occasion to leave a "wall" of anaesthetic beneath the fascia lata and just inferior to the inguinal ligament.

Drugs and dose

5-10 ml of 1% lidocaine or 0.25% bupivacaine or their equivalent (see p. 20). Epinephrine 1:200.000 may be added. If used with sciatic and femoral nerve block, 1% prilocaine is recommended on account of its lower toxicity.

Fig. 127:1.
1. Lateral cutaneous nerve of thigh
2. Femoral nerve

Figs. 127:1 and 3. Courtesy of Astra

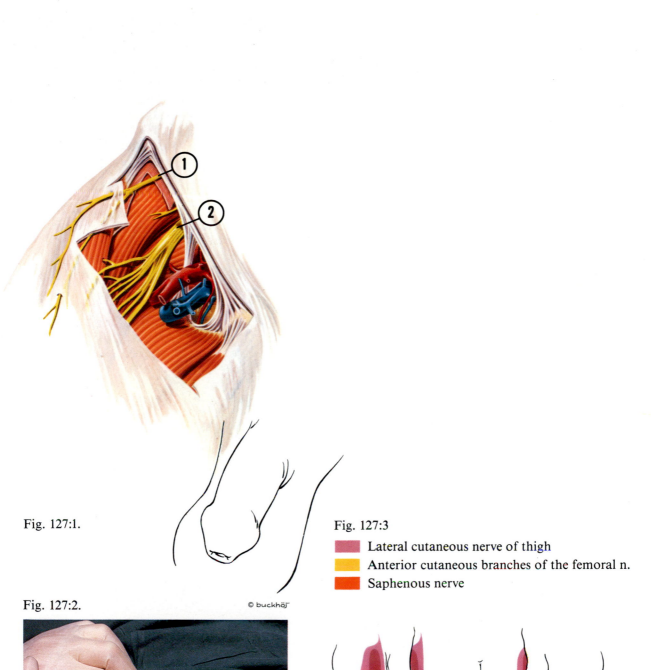

Fig. 127:1.

Fig. 127:2.

© buckhöj

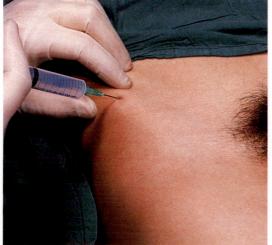

Fig. 127:3

■ Lateral cutaneous nerve of thigh
■ Anterior cutaneous branches of the femoral n.
■ Saphenous nerve

buckhöj

127

Nerve blocks at the knee

The tibial, the common peroneal and the saphenous nerves may all be blocked at the level of the knee, and will permit operations in the leg and foot or the reduction of fractures of the ankle. However, it is necessary to move the patient from the supine to the prone position to get access to all three nerves, and this may cause pain and discomfort with fractured bones.

Tibial nerve block

Anatomy
The tibial nerve is a terminal branch of the sciatic nerve. It enters the popliteal fossa between the hamstring muscles and runs close to the popliteal vessels, being medial to the artery. It leaves the fossa between the two heads of the gastrocnemius muscles (Fig. 129:2).

Patient position
Prone or lateral.

Landmarks
1. Internal and external condyles of the femur
2. Popliteal artery

Needle insertion
The needle is inserted at right angles to the skin in the middle of a line joining the condyles and medial to the popliteal artery (Fig. 129:1). Nerve stimulation will induce movement of the ankle. The nerve is 2-3 cm from the skin. If bone is contacted, withdraw the needle 5 mm.

Drugs and dose

10-15 ml of 1.5% lidocaine or 0.375% bupivacaine, or their equivalent (see p. 20). Epinephrine 1:200.000 may be added.

Fig. 129:2.
1. Sural nerve
2. Small saphenous vein
3. Medial gastrocnemius muscle
4. Popliteal vein
5. Popliteal artery
6. Medial codyle of femur
7. Tibial nerve
8. Sural artery
9. Lateral gastrocnemius muscle
10. Common peroneal nerve
11. Lateral condyle of femur

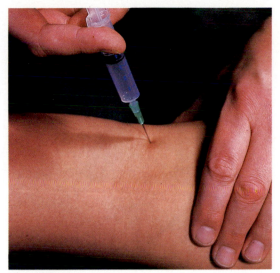

Fig. 129:1.

Fig. 129:2.

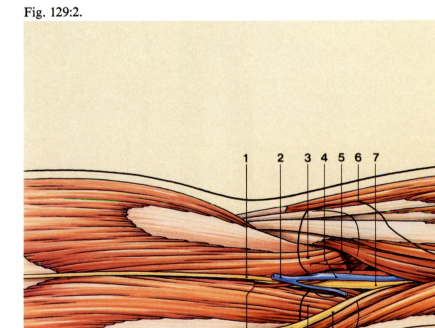

© buckhöj

129

Common peroneal nerve

Anatomy
The common peroneal nerve is also a terminal branch of the sciatic nerve. It runs between the biceps femoris tendon and the lateral head of the gastrocnemius. It winds around the head of the fibula, where it can be palpated (Fig. 131:2).

Patient position
Supine with knee slightly bent.

Landmarks
1. Head of fibula
2. Deep peroneal nerve which can be rolled on the bone

Needle insertion
Insert vertical to skin 2 cm below the head of fibula and posterior to the bone (Fig. 131:1).

Avoid eliciting paraesthesias. A nerve stimulator (p. 28) can be used and will induce movement of the toes.

Drugs and dose
5 ml of 1.5% lidocaine or 0.375% bupivacaine or their equivalent (see p. 20). Epinephrine 1:200.000 may be added.

Fig. 131:2.
1. *Biceps femoris tendon*
2. *Lateral condyle of tibia*
3. *Head of fibula*
4. *Common peroneal nerve*
5. *Deep peroneal nerve*
6. *Superficial peroneal nerve*
   (lateral cutaneous nerve of calf)

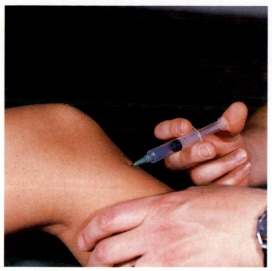

Fig. 131:1.

Fig. 131:2.

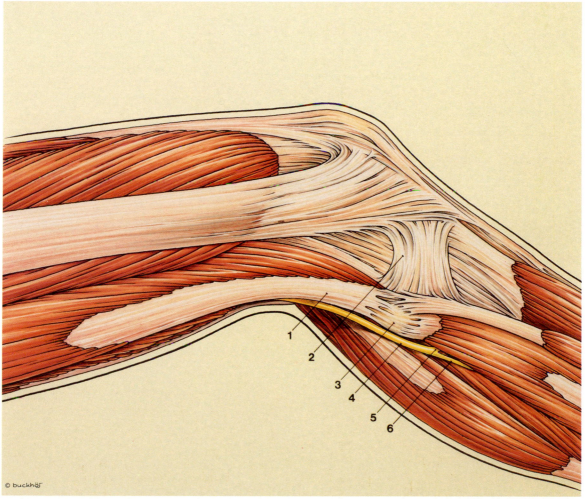

© buckhöj

Saphenous nerve

Anatomy
The saphenous nerve becomes subcutaneous at the knee and can easily be blocked by infiltration (Fig. 133:2).

Patient position
Supine, knee slightly bent.

Landmarks
Tibial tuberosity and medial head of gastrocnemius.

Needle insertion
Make a subcutaneous infiltration between the tibial tuberosity and the medial head of gastrocnemius (Fig. 133:1).

Drugs and dose
5-10 ml of 1% lidocaine or 0.25% bupivacaine or their equivalent (see p. 20). Epinephrine 1:200.000 may be added.

Fig. 133:2.
1. Saphenous nerve
2. Tibial tuberosity
3. Pes anserinus
4. Infrapatellar branch
5. Gastrocnemius muscle
6. Great saphenous vein

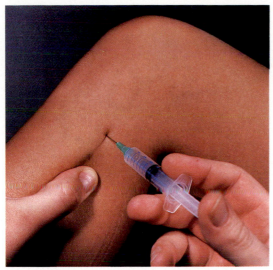

Fig. 133:1.

Fig. 133:2.

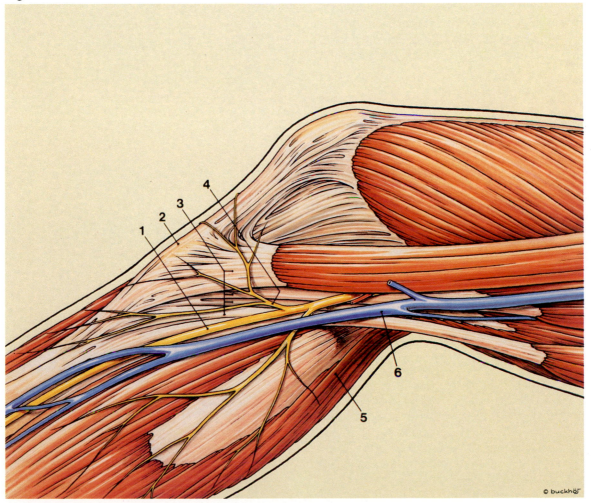

Nerve block at the ankle

Five nerves supply the foot, four of which derive from the sciatic nerve (the tibial, the superficial and deep peroneal nerves, and the sural nerve) and one from the femoral nerve (the saphenous nerve) (Fig. 135:1 and 135:4). It is important to distinguish between those nerves which supply the deep structure, (bones, joints, muscles and tendons) and those which only supply skin. The former have to be blocked beneath the deep fascia while the latter may be blocked by simple subcutaneous infiltration.

Two nerves supply the deep structures of the foot, the tibial (through its two terminal branches, the lateral and medial plantar nerves) and the deep peroneal. Both also supply areas of skin. Fortunately both are in close relationship to arteries and tendons which are usually easily identified.

Classically, ankle blocks have involved injections made above the ankle and if all five nerves are to be blocked, it is difficult to get access in supine patients, particularly for those nerves approached posteriorly, the tibial and the sural.

However, virtually complete anaesthesia of the deep structures of the foot can be obtained using the midtarsal technique of deep peroneal block described by Sharrock, Waller and Fierro, together with tibial nerve block below the medial malleolus and the ankle. This does not require the patient to be moved from the supine position.

Ankle blocks can be used alone for many types of foot surgery, or they may be combined with light general anaesthesia, especially if a tourniquet is to be used. They provide excellent operating conditions and a very valuable period of postoperative analgesia.

It is not necessary to block all five nerves in every case. This will depend on the operative site and it is frequently unnecessary to block the sural nerve or the saphenous nerve. However, if deep structures are involved, the tibial nerve and the deep peroneal nerve must be blocked beneath the deep fascia. It is not necessary or desirable to elicit paraesthesia.

Fig. 135:1.
1. Saphenous nerve
2. Long saphenous vein
3. Anterior tibial muscle
4. Deep peroneal nerve
5. Extensor hallucis longus muscle
6. Superficial peroneal nerve
7. Dorsalis pedis artery

Fig. 135:4.
1. Flexor retinaculum
2. Tibial nerve
3. Posterior tibial artery
4. Sural nerve
5. Short saphenous vein

Figs. 135:1-4. Courtesy of Astra.

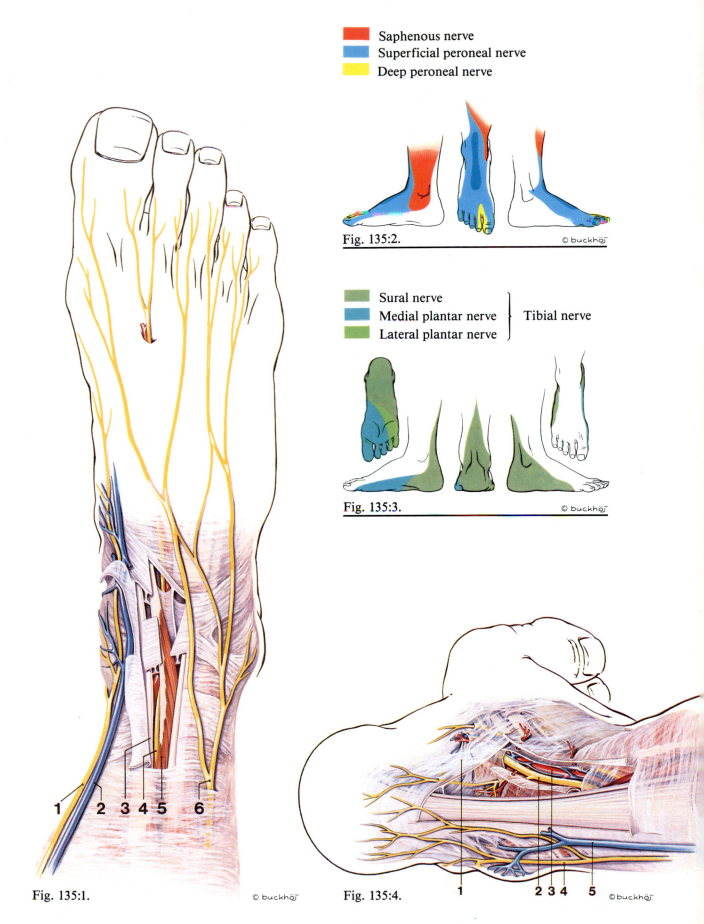

Saphenous nerve
Superficial peroneal nerve
Deep peroneal nerve

Fig. 135:2.

Sural nerve
Medial plantar nerve
Lateral plantar nerve
Tibial nerve

Fig. 135:3.

Fig. 135:1.

1   2   3   4   5   6

Fig. 135:4.

1   2   3   4   5

135

Tibial nerve block

Anatomy
At the ankle the tibial nerve runs on the posterior surface of the tibia, medial to the tendo Achillis and behind the posterior tibial artery. It passes between the medial malleolus and the flexor retinaculum, giving off the medial calcanean branches which supply the skin of the heel (Fig. 135:4). Passing forward under the malleolus, the tibial nerve divides into the medial and lateral plantar nerves which supply the deep structures and most of the skin of the sole and the plantar surfaces of the toes. The terminal branches (the plantar digital nerves) also supply the dorsal surfaces of the distal parts of the toes, including the toe-nails.

Patient position
Supine with foot externally rotated, and knee flexed.

Landmarks
1. The medial malleolus
2. The posterior tibial artery below the medial malleolus and the flexor retinaculum

Needle insertion
Palpate the artery below the malleolus and insert the needle behind it to penetrate the deep fascia and contact bone (Fig. 137:4). Inject 3-5 ml of local anaesthetic. If the artery cannot be felt, injection below and behind the medial malleolus will usually be successful.

Drugs and dose
3-5 ml of 1% lidocaine or 0.25% bupivacaine will give satisfactory blocks (Fig. 137:3). However, if postoperative analgesia is wanted, this will be more prolonged if higher concentrations are used. Because the total volume is not high, 2% lidocaine or 0.5% bupivacaine or their equivalents (see p. 20) can be used. Epinephrine 1:200.000 can be added.

Complications
See p. 138.

Deep peroneal nerve block

Anatomy
The deep peroneal nerve descends in front of the ankle in close relationship to the anterior tibial artery, which is lateral to it (Fig. 137:1). It runs with the artery, (which becomes the dorsalis pedis artery) under the extensor retinaculum to reach the dorsum of the foot. It supplies the deep structures and a small area of skin between the great and second toes and the adjacent part of the dorsum of the foot.

Patient position
Supine.

Landmarks
1. Dorsalis pedis artery
2. Tendon of extensor hallucis longus

Needle insertion
The nerve is closer to the artery than the tendon and the needle should be inserted just lateral to the artery to penetrate the deep fascia and contact bone (Fig. 137:1). Inject 3-5 ml. Some authorities inject on both sides of the artery.

Drugs and dose
1% lidocaine or 0.25% bupivacaine will give satisfactory blocks (Fig. 137:2). However, if postoperative analgesia is wanted, this will be more prolonged if higher concentrations are used. Because the total volume is not high, 2% lidocaine or 0.5% bupivacaine or their equivalents (see p. 20) can be used. Epinephrine 1:200.000 can be added.

Complications
See p. 138.

Figs. 137:1-4. Courtesy of Astra.

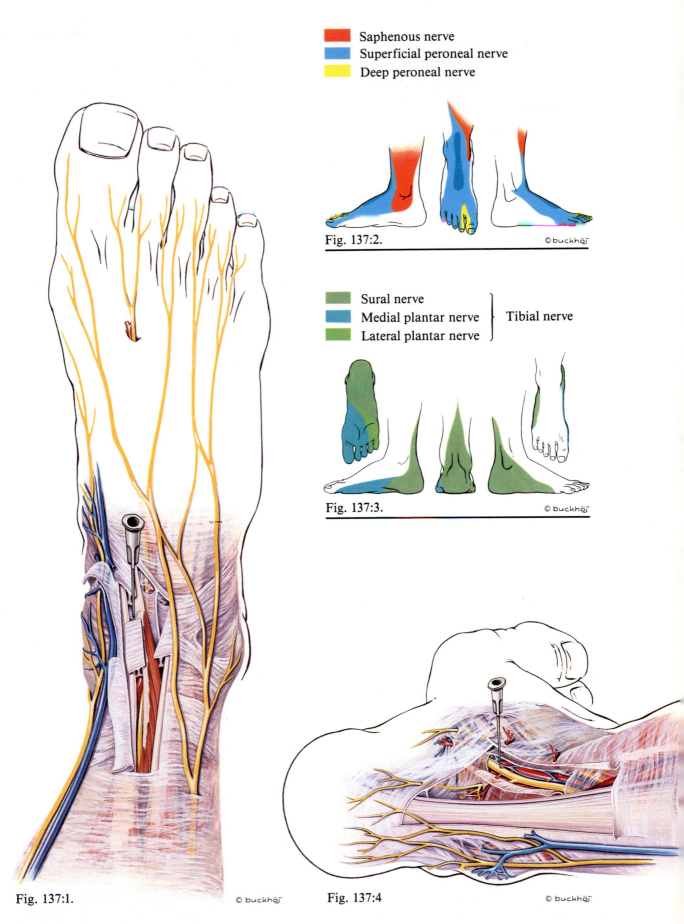

Saphenous nerve
Superficial peroneal nerve
Deep peroneal nerve

Fig. 137:2.

© buckhöj

Sural nerve
Medial plantar nerve } Tibial nerve
Lateral plantar nerve

Fig. 137:3.

© buckhöj

Fig. 137:1.

© buckhöj

Fig. 137:4

© buckhöj

137

Superficial peroneal, sural and saphenous nerve block

Anatomy

The superficial peroneal nerve pierces the deep fascia well above the ankle, in the lower third of the leg. It soon divides and its branches run anteriorly to the ankle to supply those parts of the skin of the dorsum of the foot which are not supplied by the deep peroneal and the sural nerves.

The **sural nerve** (Fig. 139:4), which, like the tibial nerve, is a terminal branch of the sciatic nerve, reaches the ankle behind the lateral malleolus and lateral to the calcaneus. It is in the superficial fascia and closely related to the small saphenous vein. It supplies the lateral border of the foot and the small toe (Fig. 139:3).

The **saphenous nerve** (Fig. 139:1) becomes subcutaneous in the thigh. It runs with the long saphenous vein along the medial border of the tibia. It passes in front of the medial malleolus and supplies the skin on the medial side of the foot as far as the first metatarsophalangeal joint.

Because these nerves are all within the superficial fascia they may easily be blocked by subcutaneous infiltration. The easiest way to do this is to encircle the ankle, at the level of the malleoli, with a ring of subcutaneous local anaesthetic. Some would avoid a complete circle, preferring two semicircles at differing levels to avoid a tourniquet effect, but it is unlikely that sufficient pressure could be generated in the subcutaneous tissues to adversely affect the circulation. 15-20 ml of 1% lidocaine or 0.25% bupivacaine with or without epinephrine is used. If it is desirable to anaesthetise these nerves individually (e.g. if sural or saphenous nerve block was not necessary) then they may be blocked as follows:

Superficial peroneal nerve block

Infiltrate subcutaneously 5 cm above the lateral malleolus, from the anterior midpoint of the leg, laterally to the level of the malleolus (Figs 139:1 and 2). 5-10 ml of lidocaine or 0.25% bupivacaine will suffice. Epinephrine 1:200.000 can be added.

Sural nerve block

Infiltrate 5 ml of local anaesthetic subcutaneously between the lateral malleolus and the tendo Achillis. (Figs. 139:3 and 4).

Saphenous nerve block

Infiltrate 5 ml of local anaesthetic around the long saphenous vein 1 cm above the medial malleolus (Figs 139:1 and 2).

Complications of ankle block

Direct trauma to nerves

Because of their small size, intraneural injections can cause considerable damage with even small volumes of injectate. Paraesthesias therefore should not be sought and, if encountered, the needle should be re-sited before making an injection.

Arterial puncture

Although arterial puncture itself is seldom damaging to the arterial wall, haematoma formation can occur and reduce the blood flow through the artery. Some care is therefore necessary in patients with peripheral vascular disease.

Figs. 139:1-4. Courtesy of Astra.

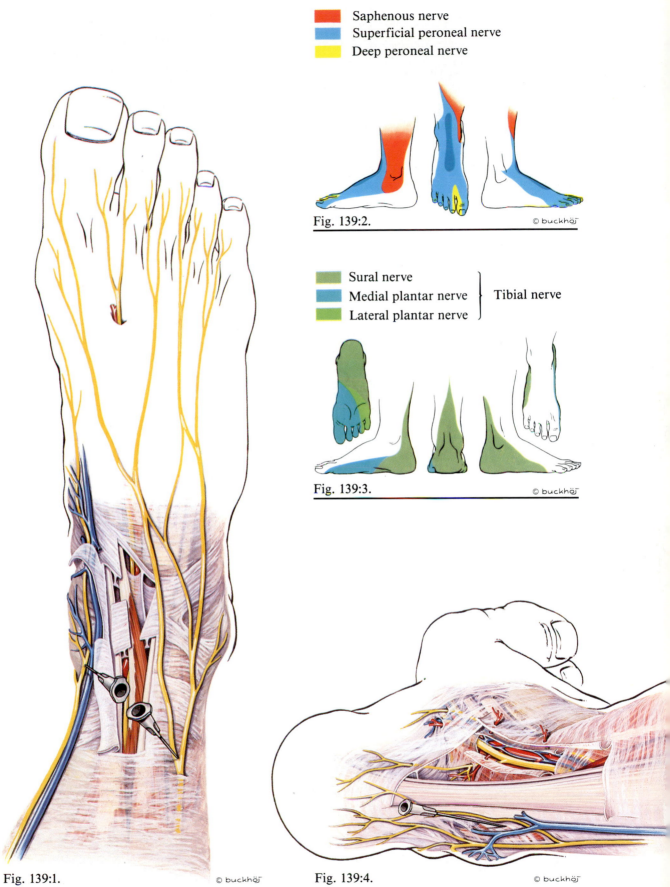

Saphenous nerve
Superficial peroneal nerve
Deep peroneal nerve

Fig. 139:2.

Sural nerve
Medial plantar nerve
Lateral plantar nerve

Tibial nerve

Fig. 139:3.

Fig. 139:1.

Fig. 139:4.

139

Digital nerve block of the toe

This is a simple and effective way of anaesthetising a toe.

Anatomy

Two nerves run on either side of each toe, a plantar and a dorsal digital nerve (Fig. 141:1).

Needle insertion

The easiest method is to insert a needle at the base of the digit to contact the proximal phalanx at its lateral point. Withdraw the needle fractionally and deposit 0.5 ml of local anaesthetic. Redirect the needle towards the dorsal part of the digit (Fig. 141:2) and inject a further 1 ml as the needle is slowly withdrawn. Repeating this on the plantar aspect of the digit (Fig. 141:3) will leave a semicircle of local anaesthetic which, when repeated on the other side of the digit, will surround the base of the toe with a complete ring of the injected drug.

Drugs and dose

4 ml of lidocaine 1% ml or its equivalent (p. 20). Epinephrine is not recommended in digital blocks.

Suggested further reading

Moore, D.C. (1975) Regional Block. C. C. Thomas, Springfield, Illinois.

Raj, P.P., Parks, R.I., Watson, T.D. and Jenkins, M.T. (1975). New single position supine approach to sciatic-femoral nerve block. Anesth. Analg. 54, 489.

Sharrock N.E., Waller, J.F., and Fiero, L.E. (1986). Midtarsal block for surgery of the forefeet. Br. J. Anaesth. 58, 37.

Winnie, A.P., Ramamurthy S. and Durani, Z. (1973). The inguinal paravascular technic of lumbar plexus anesthesia. "The 3-in-1-block". Anesth. Analg. 52, 989.

Fig. 141:1.
1. Superficial peroneal nerve
2. Deep peroneal nerve
3. Dorsal digital nerve
4. Plantar digital nerve

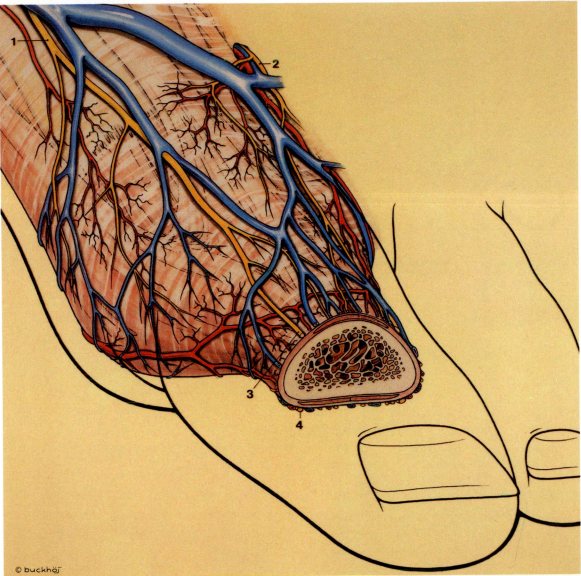

© buckhöj

Fig. 141:1.
Fig. 141:2.

Fig. 141:3.

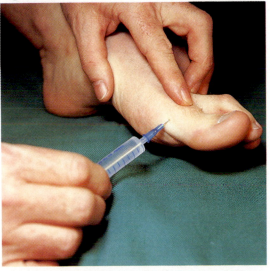

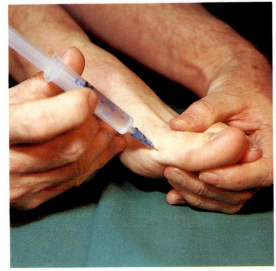

Thorax and abdomen

Intercostal nerve block

This is a simple block to perform and has uses both by itself and in conjunction with general anaesthesia. Usually several intercostal nerves must be blocked. The main indications are:

1. To provide postoperative pain relief after abdominal surgery, especially if the incision is unilateral, e.g. Kocher's incision for cholecystectomy. The 7th to 11th intercostal nerves are blocked on the appropriate side.
2. To provide postoperative pain relief after thoracotomy. In these cases the nerves may be blocked under direct vision from **within** the thorax.
3. To relieve the pain of fractured ribs. This can also assist in the treatment as it allows greater respiratory movement and painless coughing. The appropriate nerves are blocked posterior to the fractures.
4. To provide muscular relaxation and analgesia in conjunction with light general anaesthesia in abdominal surgery. In such cases the patient will be intubated but may be allowed to breathe spontaneously.

Anatomy

Each intercostal nerve derives from the ventral ramus of the corresponding thoracic spinal nerve (Fig. 145:1 and 3). These pass laterally from the paravertebral space to reach the inferior border of the ribs. They run at first between the pleura and the posterior intercostal fascia but soon reach the space between the intercostalis internus and intimus muscles (Fig. 145:2 and 4). Here they divide into two or more branches which run in the intercostal spaces supplying the muscles and skin of the thorax and abdomen. At the midaxillary line they each give off a lateral cutaneous branch which supplies the skin of the posterolateral parts of the thorax and abdomen.

The upper six nerves terminate at the sternum and their branches supply the skin of the anterior part of the thorax. The lower six nerves pass under the costal margin and supply the muscles and skin of the anterior abdominal wall. The lateral cutaneous branches pierce the intercostalis externus and divide into anterior and posterior branches to supply the skin of the lateral wall of the abdomen (as far forward as the lateral border of the rectus muscle) and the back respectively.

The cutaneous branches of the intercostal nerves communicate freely with adjacent nerves, leading to overlapping of the nerve supply. However, the major part of the skin and musculature of the abdominal wall can be anaesthetised by blockade of the 6th to 12th intercostal nerves.

In recent years there has been considerable controversy on whether there was intercommunication between adjacent intercostal spaces. At their origin the intercostal nerves, lie between the pleura and the posterior intercostal fascia (Fig. 145:2 and 4) and there is nothing to stop local anaesthetic spreading extrapleurally and affecting several adjacent nerves. Even when injected laterally at or near the costal angle, drug can reach the extrapleural space. This is made easier if ribs are fractured, when even subpleural spread can occur. These factors have led to the use of a single large volume injection in the intercostal space with the intention of causing blockade of several nerves. While this may be useful with multiple fractured ribs, the spread is unpredictable and it is better to give multiple small volume injections at the appropriate intercostal spaces.

Figs. 145:1 and 145:2.
1. *Intercostal nerve (ventral ramus)*
2. *Muscular branch*
3. *Lateral cutaneous branch*
4. *Branch to transversus thoracis muscle*
5. *Anterior cutaneous branch*
6. *Endothoracic fascia*
7. *Posterior intercostal membrane*
8. *Intercostalis externus muscle*
9. *Intercostalis internus muscle*
10. *Intercostalis intimus muscle*
11. *External intercostal membrane*

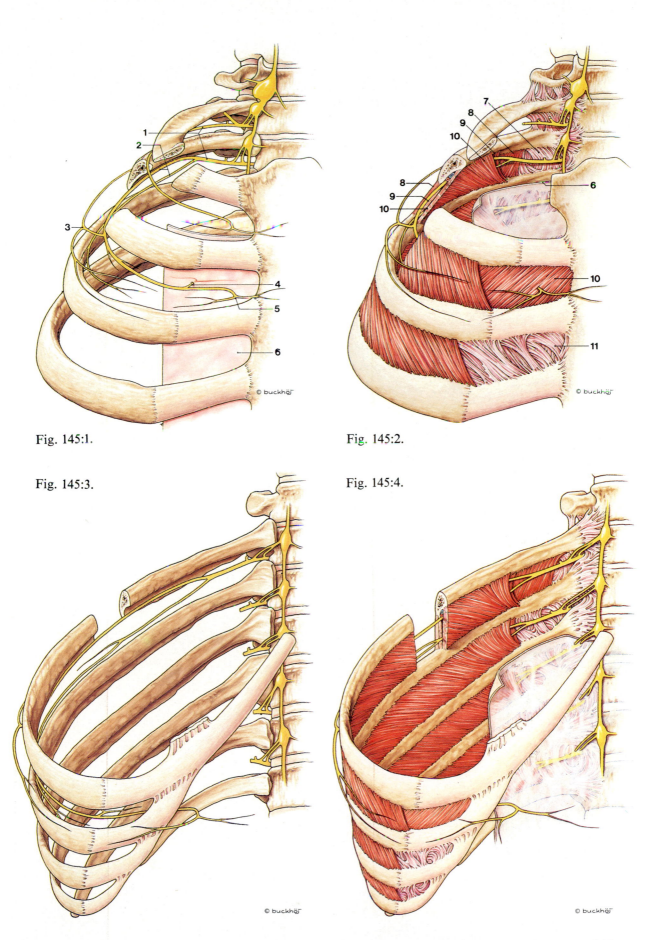

Fig. 145:1.

Fig. 145:2.

Fig. 145:3.

Fig. 145:4.

Patient position

1. Supine for blocks in the midaxillary line. This is by far the most convenient position. The arm is raised with the hand behind the head exposing the lateral thoracic wall (Fig. 147:1). Right-handed anaesthetists should face the patient's feet while blocking the right sided nerves (Fig. 147:3) and face the patient's head for the left sided nerves (Fig. 147:4). (Vice versa for left-handed anaesthetists.)

2. Lateral for unilateral blocks at the angle of the ribs.

3. Prone for bilateral blocks at the angle of the ribs.

Landmarks

1. The ribs, counting upwards from the 12th
2. The costal angles, 7-10 cm from the midline posteriorly
3. The midaxillary line

The nerves to be blocked will be determined by the indication for the block. For fractured ribs the local anaesthetic is placed close to the rib proximal to the fracture. With multiple blocks for postoperative pain relief (or as an adjunct to general anaesthesia) in abdominal surgery, the classical site for injection is at the angle of the rib, which involves the patient being in the lateral or prone position. However, drug injected into the intercostal spaces has been shown to run backwards and forwards in the spaces for several centimetres. Thus if the midaxillary line is used, the intercostal nerves, including their lateral branches, are easily blocked and the patient can remain supine.

146

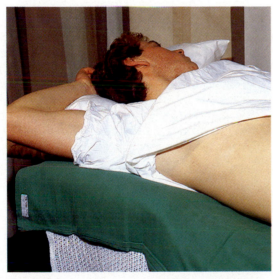

Fig. 147:1.

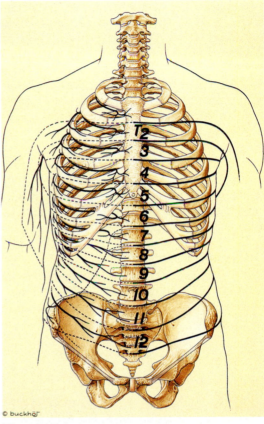

Fig. 147:2.

Fig. 147:3.

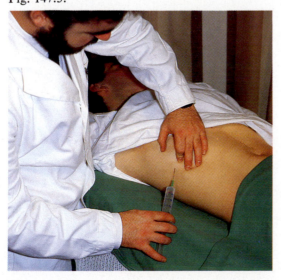

Fig. 147:4

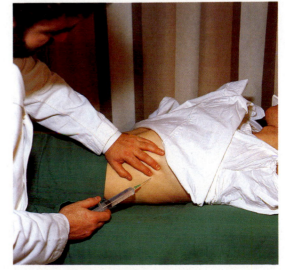

Needle insertion

Regardless of the site of injection (midaxillary or angle of the rib), the technique of needle insertion is the same. The needle point should be in close proximation to the rib if puncture of the pleura is to be avoided.

The rib is held between the second and third fingers of the non-dominant hand. The needle, attached to a syringe, is inserted between the fingers and advanced to contact the rib (Figs. 149:1 and 149:2). The needle should be directed towards the rib but tilted 20° cephalad. The needle is then "walked" down the rib until it slides under the rib, still maintaining the cephalad direction (Figs. 149:1 and 149:3). It is advanced 3 mm deep to the external surface of the rib. The anaesthetist will feel a "click" as the intercostalis externa is pierced and the needle will reach the space between internus and intimus (Fig. 149:1). 2-3 ml of local anaesthetic is injected. (An alternative method is to angle the needle almost in the plane of the rib so as to reduce the risk of pleural puncture.)

Drugs and dose

2% lidocaine, 0.5% bupivacaine or their equivalent. Epinephrine 1:200.000 may be added. Use 2-3 ml per nerve. Maximum dose 20-25 ml.

Complications

Pneumothorax

To cause a pneumothorax the needle must penetrate the pleura **and** puncture the lung itself, thus allowing sufficient air to escape into the pleural cavity and collapse the lung. Coughing and positive pressure respiration will increase the volume of air in the pleural cavity if the lung is punctured.

Provided the needle is kept in close proximity to the rib, pneumothorax is very uncommon.

Toxicity

Intercostal block gives rise to the highest plasma concentrations of local anaesthetic of the commonly used methods of regional anaesthesia. Care should therefore be taken in calculating the dose and using the appropriate drugs. Fortunately multiple bilateral blocks requiring high dosage are usually performed during a concomitant general anaesthesia and overt toxicity is unlikely. With conscious patients, the injections can be spaced out in time, e.g. over 10-15 min, and this will greatly reduce the possibility of toxicity. The diagnosis and treatment of toxicity is given on p. 22.

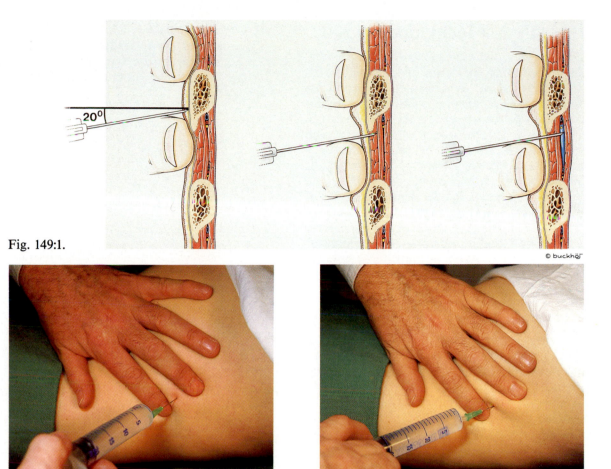

Fig. 149:1.

Fig. 149:2.

Fig. 149:3.

Interpleural local anaesthesia

It has been shown that the instillation of local anaesthetic into the pleural space (Fig. 151:1) can give excellent analgesia following upper abdominal or renal surgery involving a unilateral incision. Some success has also been obtained after thoracotomy, mastectomy and fractured ribs. The mechanism is presumably a transpleural spread of the local anaesthetic into the thoracic and intercostal nerves, and frequently it is possible to demonstrate a loss of pinprick sensation in the distribution of these nerves. The technique is easy to perform and, is when used for postoperative pain relief, free of many of the side-effects of epidural blockade such as hypotension, motor blockade and urinary retention.

Anatomy

The lower border of the lung is at the level of the 8th rib in the posterior axillary line while the pleura extends caudally as far as the 11th rib.

Patient position

Lateral with the affected side uppermost, the upper limb being flexed forward.

Needle insertion

After puncturing the skin, with a small scalpel, a Tuohy needle is inserted backwards and medially under the 8th rib, with the bevel directed cephalad (Figs. 151:1-3). The resistance of the external intercostal membrane will be felt and on puncturing this, a syringe with a freely moving plunger, containing a few millilitres of air, is attached to the needle hub (Fig. 151:4). The syringe should be above the level of the needle tip. The needle and syringe are now advanced slowly. On entering the pleural space, the negative pressure will suck in air from the syringe. The syringe is removed, an epidural catheter is fed into the pleural cavity and then the needle is removed (Fig 151:5).

Drugs and dose

Bupivacaine 20 ml of 0.5% is instilled with the patient in the lateral position. This provides on average 9 h of analgesia. The injection may then be repeated, but is said to become less effective after 24 h or so. A continuous infusion of 0.5% bupivacaine at a rate of 5-10 ml/h will maintain the blockade without repeat injections.

Complications

The obvious complication is pneumothorax, but this appear to be quite rare in published series. It may be diagnosed clinically or by chest X-ray.

Figs. 151:2-5. Photo A. Villani, Courtesy of Astra.

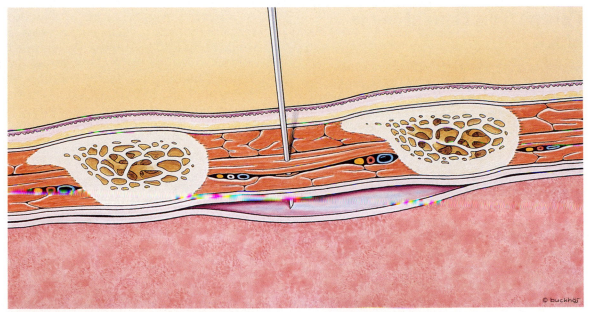

Fig. 151:1.

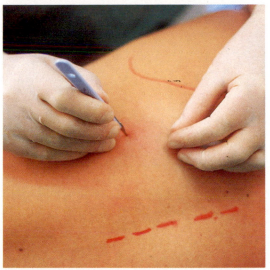

Fig. 151:2.

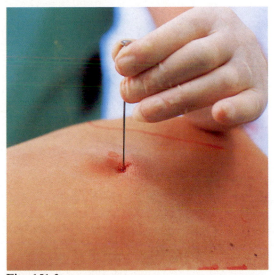

Fig. 151:3.

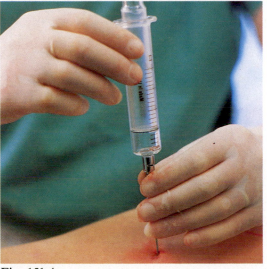

Fig. 151:4.

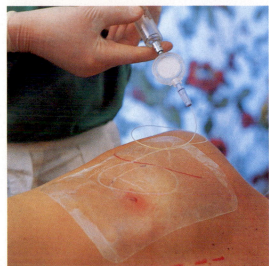

Fig. 151:5.

Paravertebral spinal nerve block

In performing paravertebral nerve block, it is necessary to contact the transverse process of the vertebra. Because of the variable angulation of the spinous processes in the thoracic region, the relationship between the spinous and transverse processes is also variable (Fig. 153:2).

In the midthoracic region T4-T9, the angulation is maximal and each spinous process is at the same level as, or just below, the transverse process of the vertebra below, i.e. T5 spinous process is at the same level as the transverse process of T6. Where angulation is less (T3 and above, T10 and below), the transverse process is at the level of the cephalad tip of the spinous process of the same vertebra.

Individual spinal nerves may be blocked as they leave the spinal canal through the intervertebral foraminae. However, it is possible to achieve blockade of several nerves with a single large volume paravertebral injection particularly in the thorax where there are no structures to inhibit the paravertebral spread of local anaesthetic. By using a catheter technique excellent analgesia can be obtained e.g. after thoracotomy.

Ideally paravertebral nerve block should be performed with radiological control because there is a risk of intrathecal or epidural injection, either as a result of the needle entering the spinal canal via an intervertebral foramina or because the dural cuff extends outwards from the canal to the paravertebral space. For post-thoracotomy analgesia, a catheter may be inserted pre-operatively and its position confirmed during the operation.

Anatomy

Spinal nerves are formed from the junction of the anterior and dorsal spinal nerve roots. These roots combine at a variable distance from the spinal cord, from within the subarachnoid space to the intervertebral foramen (Fig. 153:1). The dorsal root ganglion also lies at a variable distance from the cord and can be medial or lateral to the junction of the two roots.

As it leaves the spinal canal through the intervertebral foramen, each spinal nerve is surrounded by, and invested with, connective tissue derived from the pia arachnoid and dura mater. Thus the pia mater becomes the endoneurium of individual nerve fibres, the arachnoid becomes the perineurium investing bundles of fibres or fasciculi, and the dura is continuous with the epineurium or outside cover of the spinal nerve.

Spinal nerves vary greatly in their thickness, the largest being those to the limbs, i.e. those of the brachial and lumbosacral plexuses.

Fig. 153:1.

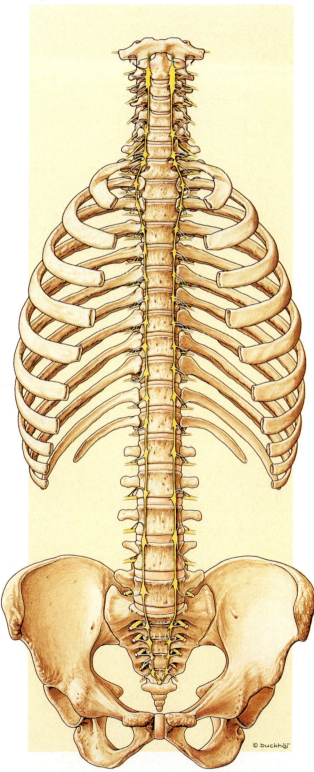

Fig. 153:2.

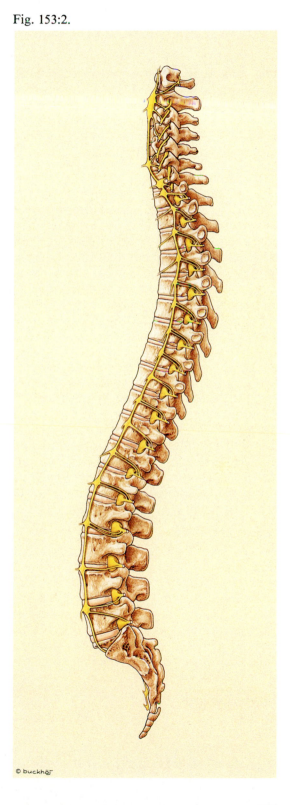

© buckhöj

© buckhöj

Thoracic paravertebral nerve block

The technique described here is for blocks between T4 and T9. Above and below this, use the lumbar technique.

Patient position

Prone with a pillow under the chest.

Landmarks

The individual spinous processes. The iliac crest is at the level of L4. The inferior rib margin 10 cm from the midline is at L2. The tip of the scapula is at T7, the spine of the scapula is at T3 (Fig. 155:1). C7 is the most prominent of the cervical spinous processes.

Needle insertion

Having identified the appropriate vertebral spinous process, and its relationship to the transverse process (See p. 152), a skin wheal is raised 3-4 cm lateral to the midline. The needle is inserted perpendicularly and should contact the transverse process 3-4 cm below the skin (Fig. 155:2). The needle is withdrawn and redirected candad so as to pass below the transverse process. 2-2.5 cm deep to the process the needle tip should be in close proximity to the spinal nerve. If bone is contacted it is likely to be the vertebral body. Paraesthesia may be encountered, and some authorities prefer to redirect the needle several times until a paraesthesia is obtained. However, it is much better to use radiological control to determine the position of the needle tip. Once a satisfactory position is obtained, a small quantity of radio-opaque dye may be injected to confirm the position and to eliminate the possibility of subarachnoid, epidural or IV injection.

Drugs and dose

5 ml of 2% lidocaine or 0.5% bupivacaine or their equivalent (see p. 20) with or without epinephrine 1:200.000 for each nerve. 0.75% bupivacaine may be preferred for a prolonged effect. If several nerves are to be blocked with a single injection (see p. 152), a catheter should be inserted and aliquots of 10-15 ml of 0.5% bupivacaine injected until the desired spread is achieved.

Complications

1. Acute toxicity if large volumes are used.
2. Trauma to individual spinal nerves.
3. Subarachnoid or epidural injection if the needle enters the spinal canal or a long dural cuff.

Lumbar paravertebral block

This is very similar to thoracic paravertebral block in the lower part of the thorax except that the needle passes above and not below the transverse process. It is important to contact the transverse process of the vertebra below the nerve to be blocked, e.g. L2 transverse process for L1 block.

Patient position

Prone with a pillow under the chest and abdomen.

Landmarks

The individual spinous processes. The iliac crest is at the level of L4. The inferior rib margin 10 cm from the midline is at L2. The tip of the scapula is at T7, the spine of the scapula is at T3. C7 is the most prominent of the cervical spinous processes.

Needle insertion

A skin wheal is raised 3-4 cm lateral to the cephalad tip of the selected spinous process. The needle is directed perpendicular to the skin and advanced 3-4 cm until it contacts the lateral process (Fig.155:3). It is then withdrawn and redirected so as to pass above the spinous process. 2-2.5 cm below deep to this it will be close to the spinal nerve. If bone is contacted it will probably be the lateral side of the vertebral body.

Paraesthesia may be elicited but it is safer and better to rely upon radiological evidence that the needle tip is correctly placed. A test dose (2 ml) of radio-opaque dye should be injected to exclude subarachnoid, epidural or IV injection.

Drugs and dose

5 ml of 2% lidocaine or 0.5% bupivacaine, with or without epinephrine 1:200.000 for each nerve. 0.75% bupivacaine may be used for prolonged blocks.

Complications

1. Acute toxicity if large volumes are used.
2. Trauma to individual spinal nerves leading to neuropathy.
3. Subarachnoid or epidural injection if the needle enters the spinal canal or a long dural cuff.

Fig. 155:1.

1. *Inferior angle of scapulae (T7)*
2. *Rib margin 10 cm from midline (L2)*
3. *Superior aspect of iliac crest (L4)*
4. *Posterior superior iliac spine (S3)*

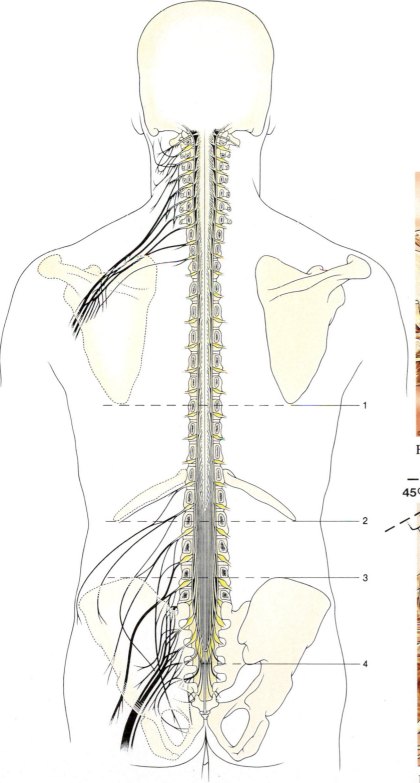

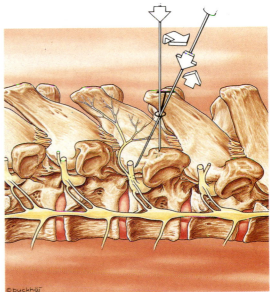

Fig. 155:2.

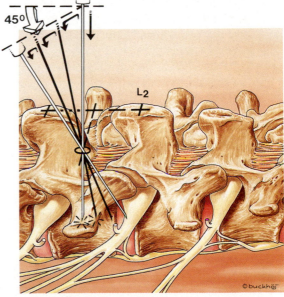

Fig. 155:3.

Trans-sacral block

Anatomy
The sacral spinal nerves do not leave the sacrum until they have divided into their anterior and posterior primary rami. The former leave the sacrum through the pelvic sacral foramina and the latter through the dorsal sacral foramina. All these foramina communicate with the sacral spinal canal (Figs. 157:2 and 157:3).

It is possible to insert a needle through a dorsal foramen and anaesthetise the corresponding sacral spinal nerve as the local anaesthetic will reach both anterior and posterior primary rami.

Patient position
Prone with pillow under the pubis.

Landmarks
1. The posterior superior iliac spine
2. The sacral cornua

A line is drawn from a point 1 cm medial to the posterior superior iliac spine, a point 1 cm lateral to the sacral cornua. This line is immediately posterior to the dorsal sacral foramina, the second being 1 cm caudad to the level of the posterior superior iliac spine and the 4th being 1 cm cephalad to the level of the sacral cornua. The foramina are each 2 cm apart.

Needle insertion
A short 22 gauge needle is used and inserted over the chosen sacral foramen. It is best to try to contact the posterior wall of the sacrum first and then to walk the needle until it can be advanced deeper into the foramen. At a depth of 1-2.5 cm (the higher foramina are deeper than the lower) the local anaesthetic is injected after preliminary aspiration (Fig. 157:1).

Drugs and dose
5 ml of 2% lidocaine or 0.5% bupivacaine or their equivalent. 0.75% bupivacaine may be used if a prolonged block is required. Epinephrine 1:200.000 may be added.

For a neurolytic blockade in the treatment of pain, 6% phenol may be used.

Complications
It is theoretically possible to reach the epidural space, and even the subarachnoid space, if a long dural cuff surrounds the nerve. This possibility should be eliminated if phenol is to be used, by using a test dose of local anaesthetic first.

Fig. 157:1.

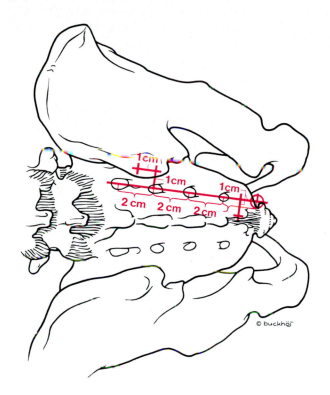

1cm 1cm 1cm
2 cm 2 cm 2 cm

© buckhöj

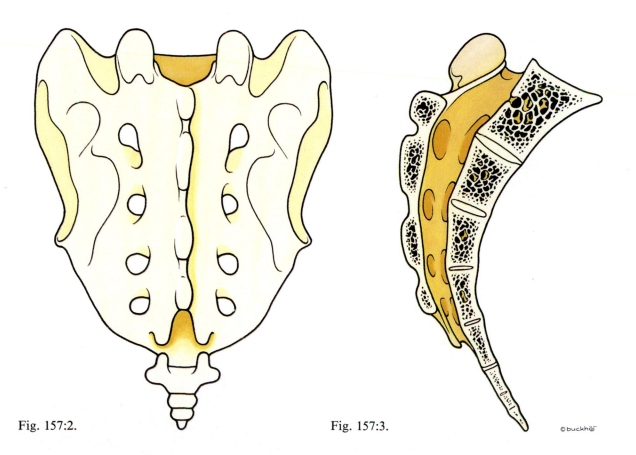

Fig. 157:2.

Fig. 157:3.

© buckhöj

Pudendal block

The major use of pudendal block is for forceps delivery. It should therefore be used by all those practising obstetrics as it eliminates the risks associated with general anaesthesia, particularly aspiration of gastric contents.

Anatomy

The pudendal nerve is derived from the 2nd, 3rd and 4th sacral spinal nerves and supplies the perineum, the introitus and the lower vagina (Fig 159:5). Before dividing into its terminal branches it runs in close proximity to the ischial spine, which is easily identified by vaginal palpation. This is therefore the ideal place to block the nerve. (Fig. 159:1 and 2).

Patient position

Lithotomy.

Landmarks

The ischial spinal and the sacrospinous ligament are identified by palpation through the vagina.

Needle insertion

The needle with syringe attached is inserted either through the vaginal wall (Fig. 159:3) or just lateral to the labia majora (Fig. 159:4) at the level of the ischial tuberosity. It is guided subcutaneously to the ischial spine by the palpating fingers in the vagina and should pierce the sacrospinous ligament, where it is in close proximity to the ischial spine (Fig. 159:1). After aspiration. The procedure is repeated on the opposite side.

If an episiotomy is to be performed, lidocaine can also be infiltrated along the line of the incision. Some obstetricians prefer to use bilateral local infiltration of the perineum for forceps delivery and omit the pudendal nerve block.

Drugs and dose

20 ml of lidocaine 1% is sufficient for bilateral pudendal block (10 ml per nerve). If 0.25% bupivacaine is used, a longer duration will be obtained which reduces the post-partum pain of perineal sutures. Epinephrine 1:200.000 may be added.

For the infiltration use lidocaine 0.5%, 10 ml for each side. Epinephrine 1:200.000 can be added and will reduce the bleeding from the episiotomy.

Complications

Because the perineum and vagina are very vascular there is a real risk of toxicity if too much local anaesthetic is injected. The recommended dose should therefore be carefully adhered to and the addition of epinephrine 1:200.000 is advisable.

During needle insertion, the rectum must be avoided by careful palpation of the needle on its way to the ischial spine.

Fig. 159:1-5. Courtesy of Astra.

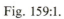
Fig. 159:1.

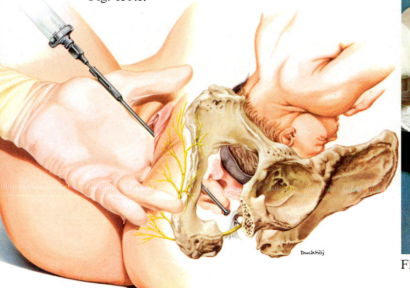

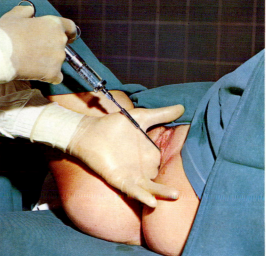
Fig. 159:2.

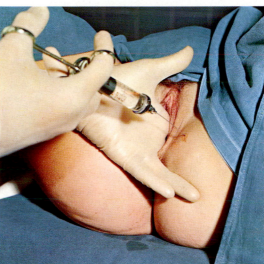
Fig. 159:3.

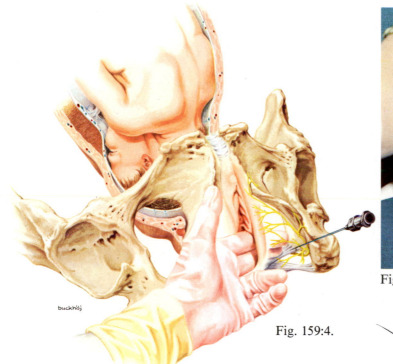
Fig. 159:4.

Fig. 159:5.

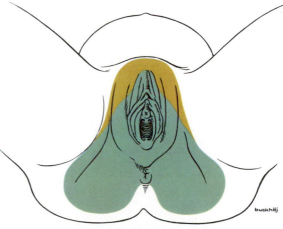

■ Indeterminate area of mixed innervation
(pudendal, ilioinguinal and
genitofemoral nn.)

■ Area of exclusive supply by the pudendal n.

159

Suggested further reading

Katz, J. and Renck, H. (1987). Handbook of Thoraco-abdominal Nerve Block. Mediglobe, Fribourg.

Reiestad, F. and Strømslaug, K.E. (1986). Intrapleural catheter in the management of postoperative pain: a preliminary report. Regional Anesth. 11, 89.

Thompson, G.E. and Moore, D.C. (1988). Celiac plexus, intercostal and minor peripheral blockade. In Neural Blockade, eds Cousins, M.C. and Bridenbaugh, P.O. Lippincott, Philadelphia, p. 503.

Central neural blockade

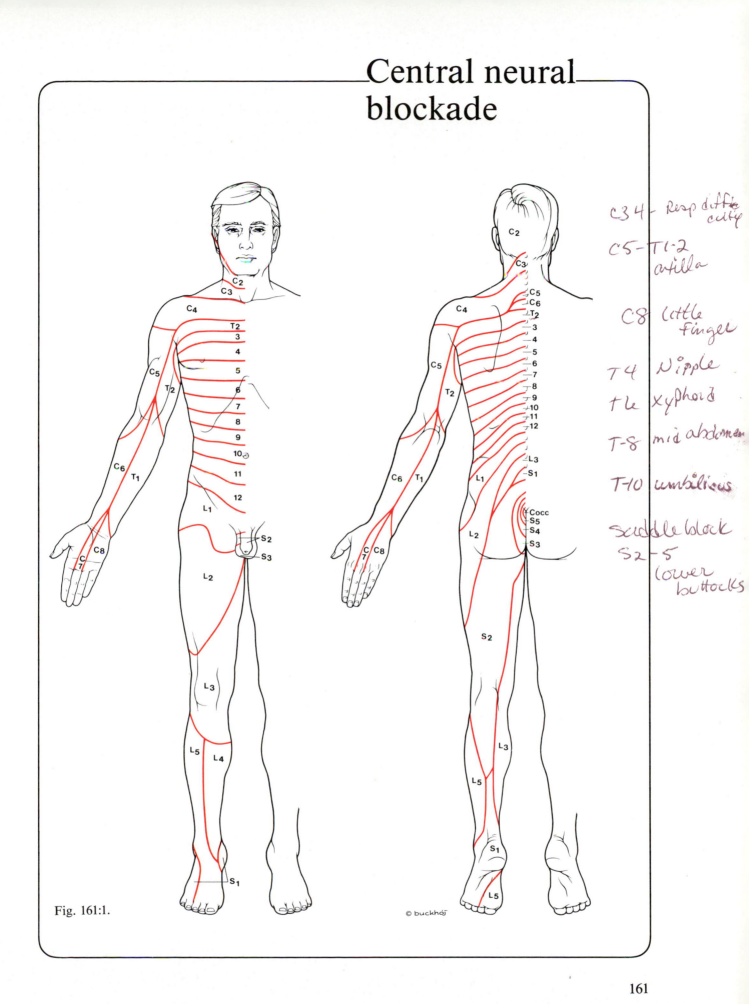

Fig. 161:1.

© buckhöj

C3 4 - Resp difficulty

C5 - T1-2 axilla

C8 little finger

T4 Nipple

T6 Xyphoid

T-8 mid abdomen

T-10 umbilicus

Saddle block S2-5 lower buttocks

Epidural blockade

The epidural space lies within the spinal canal, outside the spinal dura mater. Local anaesthetic injected into the epidural space will spread both up and down the spinal canal, blocking the spinal nerves as they run from the spinal cord to their respective intervertebral foramina.

All modalities of nerve function will be affected by epidural block, namely motor, sensory and autonomic. However, it is possible to produce a differential block by adjustment of the concentration of local anaesthetic. Unlike spinal anaesthesia, when the local anaesthesia mixes with, and diffuses in, the cerebrospinal fluid, in epidural anaesthesia the local anaesthetic must spread by volume displacement. It is often assumed that local anaesthetic escapes from the epidural space through the intervertebral foraminae and that epidural injections are therefore unpredictable in their spread due to this leakage. For both anatomical and practical reasons, however, it is best to think of the epidural space as a closed space from which lateral escape does not occur or is very limited.

Anatomy

The spinal column in which the spinal canal runs is made up of seven cervical, twelve thoracic, five lumbar and five (fused) sacral vertebrae (Fig. 163:3). These vary in their size, shape and strength depending upon the stress put upon them by the upright position. Thus the cervical vertebrae are the smallest and allow the greatest movement, while the lumbar are thick and robust with only limited movement (Fig. 163:1).

All vertebrae have a common structure (Fig. 163:2), consisting of a vertebral body anteriorly and an arch of bone posteriorly, surrounding the spinal canal. The arch consists of two pedicles anteriorly and two laminae posteriorly. At the junction of a pedicle and a lamina is the transverse process. Where the laminae meet is the spinous process.

The spinous processes vary in regard to their caudal angulation, being almost horizontal except in the mid-thoracic region, where the angulation is most marked. This is of importance when attempting to locate the epidural space between T3 and T9.

The sacral vertebrae are fused together to form the sacrum, but the epidural space can still be entered through the sacral hiatus.

Adjacent vertebrae are joined by the intervertebral discs and by the spinal ligaments. While the laminae and spinal processes are joined by ligaments, the pedicles are not. The gaps between the pedicles form the spinal foramina, through which the spinal nerves leave the spinal canal.

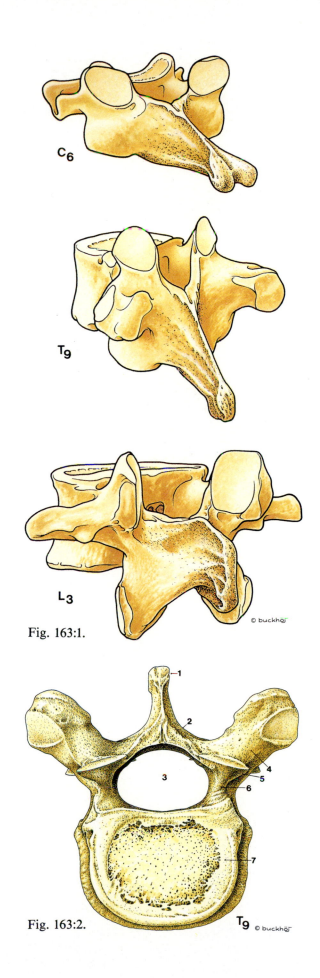

C₆

T₉

L₃

Fig. 163:1.

Fig. 163:2.

T₉

© buckhöj

© buckhöj

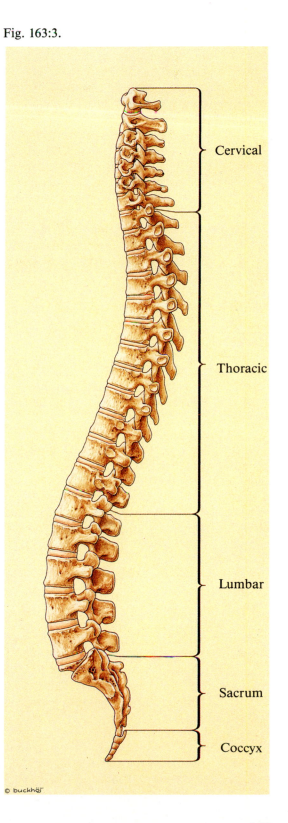

Fig. 163:3.

Cervical

Thoracic

Lumbar

Sacrum

Coccyx

© buckhöj

To reach the epidural space, the needle must pass through the supraspinous ligament, the intraspinous ligament and finally the ligamentum flavum, which joins adjacent laminae and is the thickest and toughest of the ligaments (Fig. 165:2).

The epidural space theoretically extends from the foramen magnum to the coccyx (Fig. 165:3). The spinal dura mater runs from the foramen magnum and ends around the first or second sacral vertebra. Although usually considered as a single layer of connective tissue, the spinal dura is a two-layered structure, the outer layer of which is closely applied to the wall of the spinal canal covering the bones, the discs and the ligaments which make up the canal (Figs. 165:1 and 165:2). This layer is often considered to be periosteum, but it not only covers bone but also ligaments and is easily stripped from them (unlike periosteum). In the cervical region the two layers are adherent from C1-C3.

The spinal cord runs from the brain to the level of L1/L2, while the inner layer of the dura mater ends at S1/S2 (Fig. 165:3).

Apart from spinal nerves, the epidural space contains fat, and blood vessels running to and from the vertebrae, the spinal cord, the meninges and the spinal nerves.

The epidural space can be entered anywhere in its length from the C3-4 interspace to the sacral hiatus at S4-5. Because the spinal cord ends at L1-2, the commonest point of entry is the lower lumbar region. The nerves of the cauda equina all enter the epidural space at the termination of the internal layer of spinal dura, i.e. at S1-2. Thus a lumbar approach can easily block all the sacral nerves while at the same time local anaesthetic can ascend to block the thoracic segments.

However, there are advantages to entering the epidural space at levels other than the lumbar, in order to produce discrete bands of anaesthesia at the appropriate height. Thus epidural block can be cervical, thoracic, lumbar or sacral (caudal).

Spinal nerves supply specific dermatomes in the body and different upper levels of block are required for different operations as follows:

Upper abdominal	T5-6
Lower abdominal	T8-9
Lower limb	T12
Perineal	S1
Bladder	T10
Kidney	T8

Fig. 165:1.
1. Arachnoid mater
2. Subdural space
3. Dura mater (inner layer)
4. Dura mater (Outer layer)
5. Ligamentum flavum
6. Pia mater
7. Subarachnoid space
8. Epidural space
9. Dorsal root ganglion
10. Periosteum
11. Posterior longitudinal ligament

Figs. 165:2
1. Posterior longitudinal ligament
2. Periosteum
3. Nerve root
4. Subarachnoid space
5. Epidural space
6. Pia mater
7. Arachnoid mater
8. Subdural space
9. Subarachnoid septum
10. Dura mater (inner layer)
11. Dura mater (outer layer)
12. Ligamentum flavum
13. Ligamentum denticulatum
14. Dorsal nerve root
15. Ventral nerve root
16. Dorsal root ganglion
17. Spinal nerve

Fig. 165:3
1. Vertebra
2. Periosteum
3. Epidural space
4. Dura mater
5. Subdural space
6. Arachnoid mater
7. Subarachnoid space
8. Pia mater

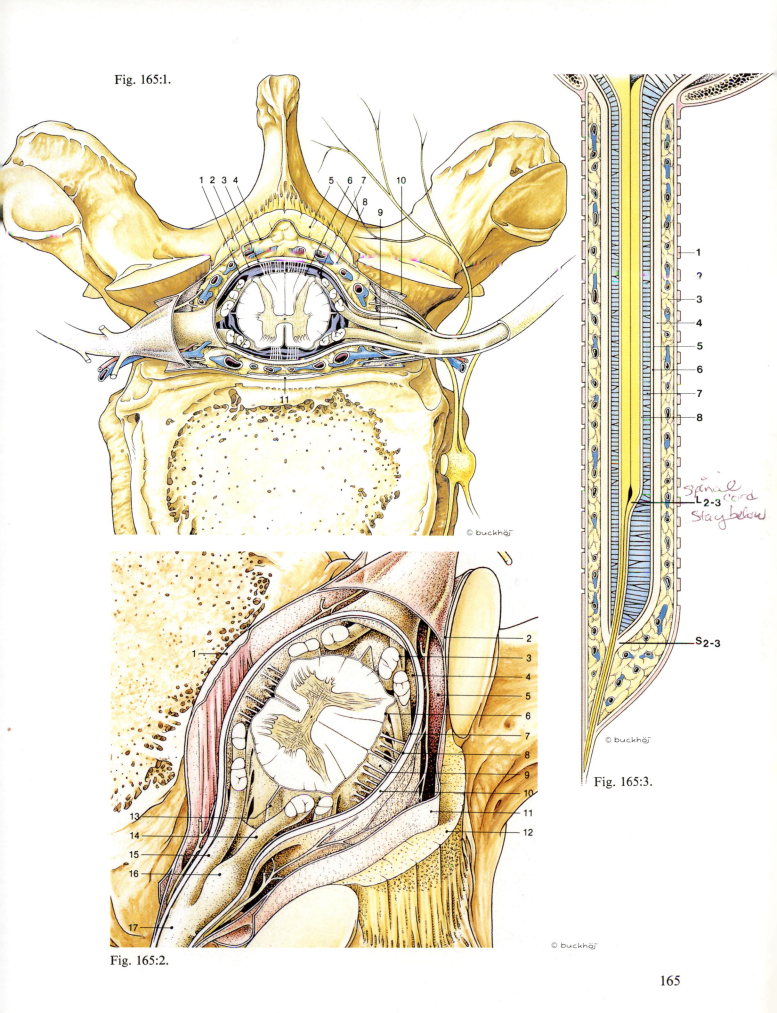

Fig. 165:1.

Fig. 165:2.

Fig. 165:3.

spinal cord stay below

L 2-3

S 2-3

165

The autonomic nervous system

The preganglionic sympathetic nerves arise from the 14 spinal segments from T1-L2, while the sacral parasympathetics derive from S2-4 (Fig. 167:1. Widespread blockade of autonomic nerves can have profound physiological effects.

Fig. 167:1
1. Pharyngeal plexus
2. Superior vagal ganglion
3. Inferior vagal ganglion
4. Coeliac ganglion
5. Coeliac plexus
6. Mesenteric ganglion
7. Superior hypogastric plexus
8. Inferior hypogastric plexus
9. Superior cervical ganglion
10. Middle cervical ganglion
11. Stellate ganglion
12. Coeliac ganglion
13. Superior mesenteric ganglion
14. Inferior mesenteric ganglion
15. Superior hypogastric plexus

Parasympathetic   **Sympathetic**

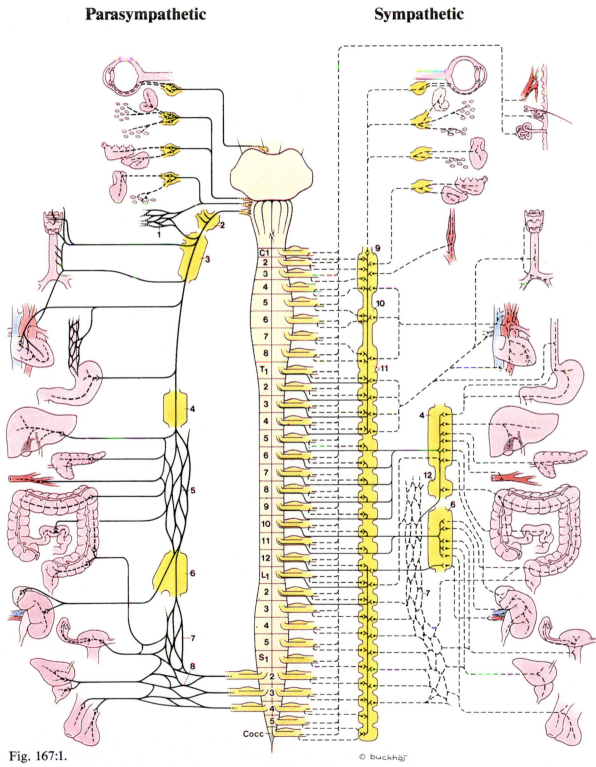

Fig. 167:1.

© buckhöj

167

Equipment

Because the spinal canal is being entered and subarachnoid puncture can occur accidentally, it is essential that all aseptic and antiseptic precautions are taken. The anaesthetist should wear sterile rubber gloves and work with a sterile pack. Because catheter techniques are commonly used to extend the duration of the block, Tuohy needles (16 or 18 gauge) with a Huber point are the most popular.

The pack should also contain:

1. Syringes. If the loss of resistance technique (see p. 170) is being used, the plunger of the syringe should move easily and without resistance within the barrel.
2. Needles. Large for drawing up fluid from ampoules and small for intradermal injection.
3. Ampoules of local anaesthetic and saline.
4. Stylet for making a hole in the skin before inserting the Tuohy needle.
5. Swabs, lotion pot and sterile drapes for preparing the skin.
6. Epidural catheter and bacterial filter.

Patient position

1. Lateral with spine fully flexed (Fig. 169:2)
2. Sitting with feet on stool and bending forward (Fig. 169:3)

Patient preparation

Epidural blocks should only be performed where full anaesthetic facilities are available. A standard anaesthetic machine and all resuscitative equipment and drugs must be at hand. All anaesthetists performing epidural blocks should be able to diagnose acute generalised toxicity and total spinal anaesthesia quickly, should they occur. Treatment is simple and effective, but must be applied without delay (see p. 22).

An intravenous infusion should be set up as the first step. Blood pressure and heart rate should be recorded and many would insist that the electrocardiogram be displayed. The patient should be positioned as described above.

The patient's back is prepared with an appropriate antiseptic solution as for a surgical operation, and sterile drapes applied.

Lumbar epidural blockade

Midline approach

Landmarks

The bony landmarks are palpated. The iliac crest is felt at the level of the L4 vertebra (Fig. 169:1).

The L2-L3 and L3-L4 interspaces are those most commonly used.

Needle insertion

An intradermal wheal is raised with local anaesthetic exactly over the chosen interspace. Subcutaneous infiltration may also be used.

A large sharp needle or a stylet is then pushed through the skin to allow easy penetration with the epidural needle.

Holding the skin firmly over the spinous process with the index and middle fingers of one hand. The epidural needle is inserted in the middle of the interspace at right angles to the skin. The skin should not be allowed to move, otherwise the needle may be inserted too far laterally.

The needle is advanced until it is firmly engaged in the interspinous ligament. It now has to penetrate the ligamentum flavum to reach the epidural space (Fig. 171:1). The stylet is withdrawn.

Lateral or paramedian approach

Most anaesthetists prefer to use the midline approach, particularly in the lumbar and lower thoracic region. Some, however, maintain that a slightly lateral insertion is easier, and this is true in the midthoracic region, where the spinous processes are acutely angled (see p. 163).

Needle insertion

The needle is inserted about 1-1.5 cm lateral to the midline and on a level with the upper border of the spinous process below the chosen interspace. Thus the needle is not only more lateral but also inferior to the midline insertion (Figs. 169:4 and 169:5). It is aimed upwards and inwards to penetrate the ligamentum flavum in the midline and should not therefore contact the spinous process. If bone is contacted, it will probably be the lamina of the vertebra, and the needle must be redirected so that it enters and penetrates the ligamentum flavum.

Fig. 169:1. Courtesy of Astra.

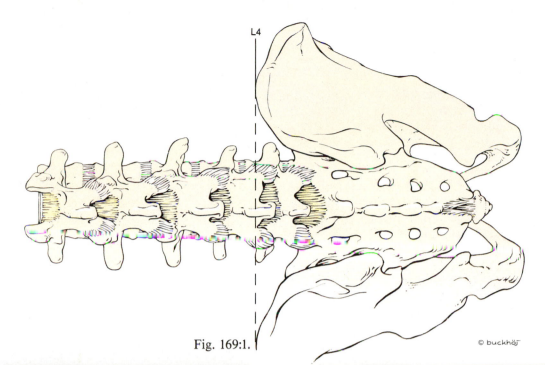

L4

Fig. 169:1.

© buckhöj

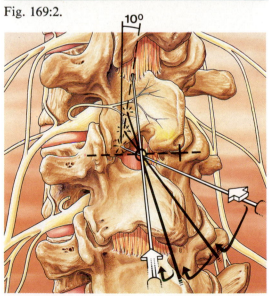

Fig. 169:2.

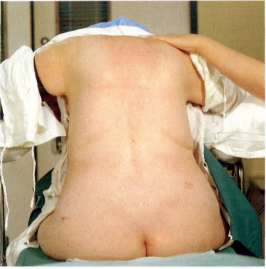

Fig. 169:3.

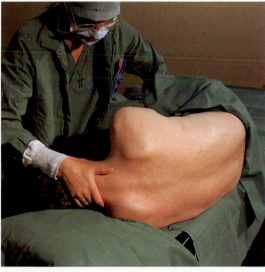

10°

Fig. 169:4.

© buckhöj

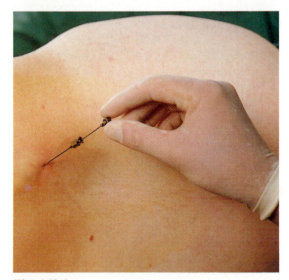

Fig. 169:5.

Identification of the epidural space

Loss of resistance technique
The commonest method used is the loss of resistance technique. There are many variations of this technique, some using the hands and others mechanical aids.

A syringe containing saline or air is attached to the needle lying in the interspinous ligament. Injection will be found to be difficult or impossible. The most difficult part of the technique to learn is the control of the advancing needle, which must not penetrate the epidural space beyond the needle bevel. The position of the hands and fingers on the needle and syringe are critical.

The index finger of the non-injecting hand may be held firmly against the patient's back to act as a resistance to sudden forward movement. The thumb and middle finger hold the needle hub (Fig. 171:1).

Alternatively the dorsum on the non-injecting hand is placed on the patient's back and the fingers can be turned back to hold the needle at its hub. The hand thus acts as an ''opponens'' to the advancing syringe and needle (Fig. 171:2).

This may even be exaggerated so that the hand grasps the lower end of the syringe (Fig. 171:3).

Where advancement of the needle is relatively easy, continuous pressure on the syringe plunger can be used, care being taken that the needle is pushed through the ligamentum flavum slowly and without a sudden forward movement, which could lead to penetration of the dura mater.

As the needle is advanced, pressure is maintained on the plunger, noting the increased resistance of the ligamentum flavum. At the moment of entering the epidural space, saline or air can be injected with great ease.

The flow of fluid (or air) from the syringe as the needle enters the epidural space pushes the dura away from the needle point (Figs. 171:5 and 171:6).

Mechanical aids include the Macintosh balloon, an intravenous infusion and a spring-loaded (Evans) syringe. These allow two-handed advancement of the needle (which is helped by a winged needle) and the immediate identification of the epidural space as the resistance to injection disappears.

''Hanging drop'' technique
The negative pressure that is often found within the epidural space is the basis for the ''hanging drop'' technique. A winged needle can be used and it is advanced with both hands. A drop of fluid is placed at the end of the needle after engaging the interspinous ligament (Fig. 171:4). When the ligamentum flavum is penetrated the drop of fluid is sucked into the epidural space, and correct identification of the space can be confirmed by injection of fluid or air without resistance.

When a blunter needle is preferred or the ligaments are difficult to penetrate, then an intermittent technique can be used. Both hands push on the needle in a controlled way and the resistance to injection is tested after every millimetre of advancement.

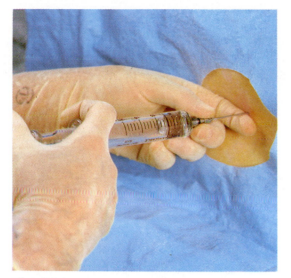

Fig. 171:1.

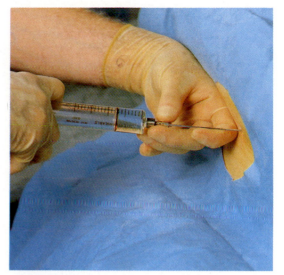

Fig. 171:2.

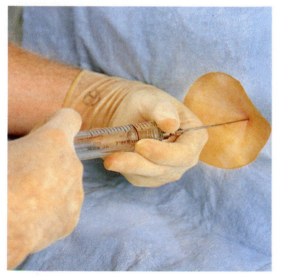

Fig. 171:3.

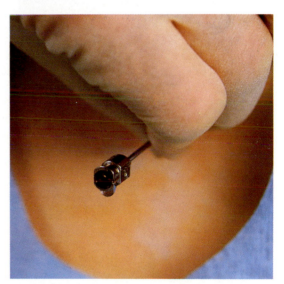

Fig. 171:4.

Fig. 171:5.

Fig. 171:6.

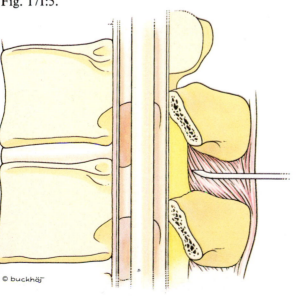

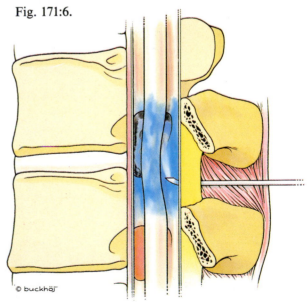

Catheter technique

If a prolonged nerve block is required, a plastic catheter can be introduced through the needle (Fig. 173:1) so that repeated injections can be made to provide a continuous epidural block for the duration of surgery and, if required, into the postoperative period. This, of course, also applies to epidural block used for relief of pain in labour.

A plastic catheter with appropriate (5 cm) distance markings is used. It is passed through the needle and into the epidural space.

The catheter is rolled in one hand to prevent it falling into an unsterile area.

A slight resistance is felt as the catheter passes through the tip of the needle, when the second distance mark will just be visible at the hub (Fig. 173:2).

By turning the needle, the Huber point can be directed cephalad or caudad. The catheter can therefore be advanced in either direction.

About 5 cm of catheter is advanced into the epidural space, when the third distance mark will be at or near the needle hub (Fig. 173:3).

The needle is then withdrawn carefully without removing the catheter, which is gently pushed forward as the needle is being retracted.

The needle is completely removed from the patient.

There are several different designs of catheter available. Some have a single terminal opening, while others have up to three lateral holes. Some are supplied with a stylet. Most are somewhat rigid at their tip and can penetrate the thin wall of an epidural vein. All are provided with a means of connecting the proximal end of the catheter to a syringe.

A bacterial filter can be attached to the end of the catheter so that all fluid injected is sterile.

Water-resistant strapping is used to keep the catheter in place.

All injections can now be made near the patient's head.

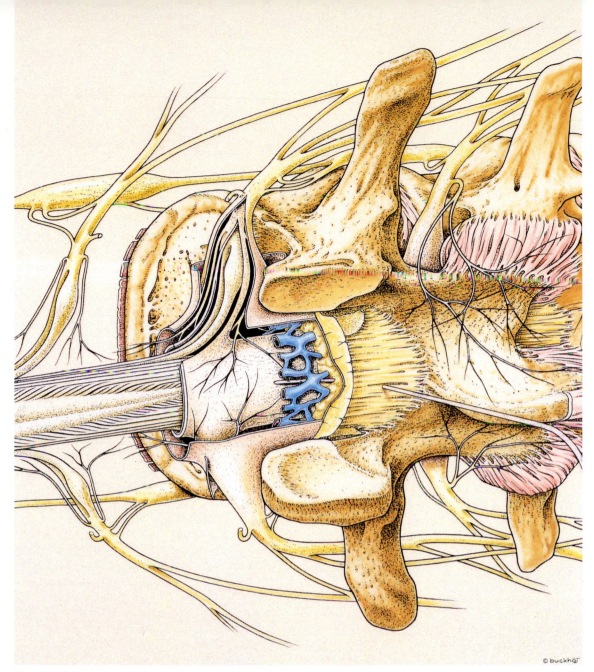

Fig. 173:1.

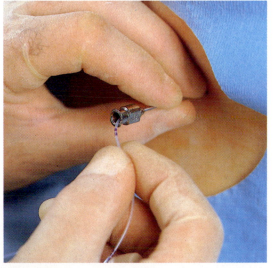

Fig. 173:2.

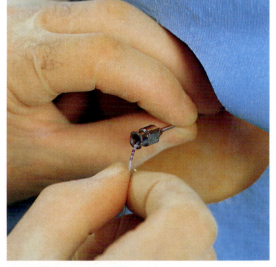

Fig. 173:3.

Drugs and dose

Test dose
Before injecting the chosen dose of drug, many anaesthetists prefer to inject a small test dose to eliminate the possibility of the needle or catheter being either in a vein, or within the subarachnoid space.

The amount of drug used as a test dose and the time allowed must be adequate to show the effects of incorrect placement. Thus 4-5 ml of drug injected into the subarachnoid space and left for 5 min will give an easily detected spinal block, whereas 2 ml left for 2 min might well not do so. 2 ml of a hyperbaric spinal solution will show most quickly that a subarachnoid injection has been made, but will have very little effect in the epidural space, unlike say 5 ml of 2% lidocaine or 0.5% bupivacaine, which may produce a block over several spinal segments. If the needle or catheter is lying within a vein, even 5 ml may be insufficient to cause systemic effects unless epinephrine (0.1 mg, i.e. 0.1 ml of 1:1.000 solution) is added and the heart rate and arterial pressure are measured before and after injection. **It is important that if a test dose is used, a negative result should not be taken as absolute proof of correct placement**. Care must still be taken while injecting the main dose. If a test dose has been given through the needle, a further test dose should be given after insertion of the catheter.

Main dose
Many drugs can be used for epidural block (Table 21:1). Because of the size and thickness of the coverings of the spinal nerves, drugs must be used in high concentration for complete nerve blockade, though weaker solutions may be used for pain relief; this is especially so when the pain is mediated through autonomic nerves, as with the pain of uterine contractions during labour.

The volume to be used (Table 174:1) will depend upon the required height of blockade and the general condition of the patient.

A common misconception is that the spread within the epidural space is linear related to the volume injected, i.e. 20 ml will involve twice as many spinal nerves as 10 ml. This is not so, because of the variability in the potential volume of the epidural space at different levels in the spinal column, and to the erratic spread of the first 5-10 ml of injectate. The last 10 ml of a 20-ml injection is likely to "fill out" the space where local anaesthetic has already reached, rather than spread to a higher level. Thus a 20-ml injection will produce a more profound and longer lasting nerve block, but will be only a few segments higher, than a 10-ml injection. There is no evidence that posture plays any part in the spread of local anaesthetic solutions in the epidural space.

The simplest approach to dosage is to plan on injecting rather more than is thought necessary to block nerves to the required level. Thus failure to achieve an adequate height will be greatly reduced and more prolonged blockade will result. Unduly high blocks are uncommon and if properly managed will cause little upset to patients unless they are either very old or very ill. With a catheter, dosage can be varied at will according to the response to the initial injection.

Because the total dose of the drug is likely to cause toxic effects if given rapidly into an epidural vein, **it is important to inject slowly** (10 ml/min) even though the test dose gave a negative result. An alternative approach is to inject the local anaesthetic in small aliquots, e.g. 5 ml every 5 min until the necessary height of blockade is achieved.

Table 174:1.
Volumes used for lumbar epidural blockade

Operation	Volume (ml)
Lower abdominal	15-20
Upper abdominal	15-25
Lower limb & perineal	10-15
Pain relief in labour	6-10
Postoperative pain relief	6-10

Complications

Misplacement of needle or catheter

The anaesthetist must ensure that the needle tip or the catheter is in the epidural space. If the catheter has been incorrectly inserted and does not lie within the spinal canal, then no nerve block will result from the injection of local anaesthetic. This possibility must be entertained if there is no evidence of a nerve block within 15-20 min. The most likely position of the catheter in such a case is the sacrospinalis muscle, lateral to the spinous process. This can occur particularly in obese patients. The anaesthetist can be misled by the ease of injection, since a loss of resistance can occur when the needle deviates laterally from the interspinous ligament and reaches the muscular compartment.

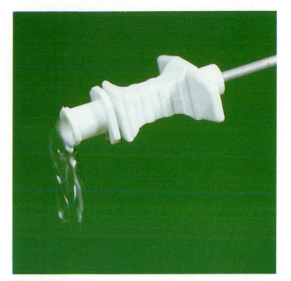

Fig. 175:1.

Dural tap

Most dural taps are due to an uncontrolled sudden forward movement of the needle as the ligamentum flavum is penetrated. Dural tap will be diagnosed by removing the syringe and observing cerebrospinal fluid (CSF) escaping from the needle (Fig. 175:1). CSF may be distinguished from the fluid used in the syringe by its temperature or by the presence of glucose. If the subarachnoid space has been entered, the escape of CSF through the large bore needle is usually so copious that there is little doubt as to the true position of the needle. A spinal headache is liable to result (see below).

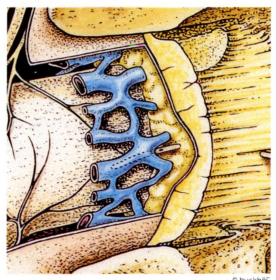

Fig. 175:2.

Intravenous placement

Penetration of an epidural vein by the needle is easy to detect as blood flows freely from the needle hub. In such a case the needle must be withdrawn and the procedure repeated at the same or an adjacent vertebral interspace.

Intravascular placement of a catheter, however, may be much more difficult to diagnose. Catheters advanced through the needle can penetrate vein walls (Fig. 175.2) and this must be checked before injecting large quantities of local anaesthetic. Simple aspiration may reveal the intravenous placement (Fig. 175:3) but this is not totally reliable as the negative pressure applied may suck the vein wall against the end of the catheter and obstruct it. It is best to lower the protruding end below the patient's spine and allow any blood to escape by gravity. If frank blood is seen, the catheter must be removed and reinserted. If blood-stained fluid is seen, the catheter or needle may or may not be

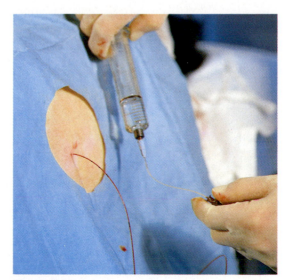

Fig. 175:3.

in a vein. A test dose as described above may then be useful in determing the location of the catheter or needle.

Hypotension

Widespread sympathetic blockade can cause a reduction in peripheral resistance due to vaso-dilatation. Because the venous capacitance is also increased, any impediment to venous return (e.g. head-up posture or caval occlusion) will cause a fall in cardiac output.

Hypotension may also be contributed to by hypovolaemia or caval occlusion, both of which require a degree of vasoconstriction to maintain a normal arterial pressure.

Sudden severe hypotension during epidural block in a conscious patient is usually due to vaso-vagal fainting. This is accompanied by pallor, bradycardia, nausea, vomiting and sweating. Patients may suffer a transient vagal cardiac arrest and can develop signs of coronary insufficiency. Consciousness will be lost during this period of arrest. This type of hypotension is not seen in patients given a concomitant general anaesthetic. Although a general anaesthetic enhances the hypotensive effects of an epidural block, the decrease in arterial pressure is not precipitate and not accompanied by vagal activity with marked bradycardia.

Treatment

If posture or caval occlusion is thought to be a factor, the patient should be repostured without delay, e.g. left lateral and head down.

Because vasodilatation is the trigger to most hypotensive episodes, it is logical to give a vasopressor (see p. 23) which will usually act rapidly and effectively. Overdosage causing **hyper**tension is to be avoided. In late pregnancy the effect of vasopressors on uterine blood flow is often feared, but an adverse effect on the foetus is unlikely if overshoot hypertension is avoided, whereas prolonged hypotension will be deleterious to the foetus.

Fluids are of use if there is evidence of hypovolaemia, but they should be backed up with vasopressors if the arterial pressure is not rapidly restored.

Atropine may be used for severe bradycardia, but vasopressors with both α- and β-receptor activity, e.g. ephedrine, will increase the heart rate satisfactorily by themselves.

Acute generalised toxicity

Because epidural block often requires large amounts of local anaesthetic, toxic reactions can occur and constant vigilance is required. The use of aspiration before injection and a test dose (provided epinephrine is added) will help prevent these reactions. Slow injection of the main dose is also essential. The symptoms, signs and treatment of toxic reactions are described on p. 22.

Total spinal anaesthesia

If by accident an excessive amount of local anaesthetic is injected into the subarachnoid space, a high or total spinal anaesthetic will ensue. This will involve widespread paralysis with respiratory arrest, severe hypotension and, if there is substantial cranial spread, unconsciousness. All these will appear within a few minutes of the injection.

Treatment is by artificial ventilation and vasopressor support of the circulation. Though alarming, total spinal block can be effectively treated if the diagnosis is made promptly.

Neurological damage
See p. 25.

Headache

Post-lumbar puncture headache can be severely debilitating and is due to leakage of CSF through puncture hole (caused by the needle) in the dura mater. Thus the size of the hole is important and this will depend upon the size of the needle, the direction of the bevel and whether or not mutiple holes were made in the dura. It is also seems to depend upon the patients age, younger patients being more affected than older ones.

The headache has distinct clinical features, being clearly related to posture in that it is worst when sitting and standing and relieved by lying down. It usually starts on the first postoperative day but may be delayed until the third day. Untreated it may take several days to disappear.

Treatment

Oral analgesics can be used if the headache is not severe, but more aggressive treatment is needed if it persists or is clearly incapacitating the patient. This involves the use of a "blood patch" i.e. the epidural injection of the patients own blood. An epidural needle is inserted into the same or an adjacent intervertebral space as was used for the spinal anaesthetic. 10-15 ml of the patients blood is withdrawn and injected (without addition of an anti-coagulant) into the epidural space. This causes an immediate increase in CSF pressure (with relief to the headache) and stops further CSF leakage. The injected blood will clot and remain in the epidural space for several days. If after treatment the headache recurs the blood patch may be repeated.

Fig. 177:1.

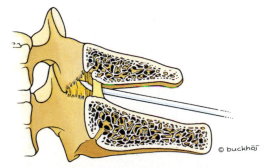

Cervical epidural block

This is very occasionally used to provide analgesia in chronic pain states, though it has been used for thoracic, thyroid and breast surgery. It has also been used for microsurgical operations on the upper limb. Access to the cervical epidural space is relatively easy, but great care must be taken to avoid direct trauma to the spinal cord. The C7-T1 interspace is the widest and easiest space to use.

Anatomy
The cervical spinous processes are not angulated and a horizontal approach is indicated (Fig. 177:1).

The epidural space is obliterated for a variable distance in the upper cervical spine (usually between the foramen magnum and C2). Thus the upper level of block will also be somewhat variable. The ligamentum flavum is relatively thin and will be reached quite superficially.

Patient position
1. Lateral with a small pillow under the head and the neck flexed.
2. Sitting up with the neck flexed.

Landmarks
Spinous process of C7. This is the most prominent of the spinous processes in the neck.

Needle insertion
The needle should be advanced with the greatest care. The usual loss of resistance will be easily appreciated. It is advised that only anaesthetists with considerable experience of lumbar epidural block should undertake this procedure.

Drugs and dose
A test dose is advisable (see p. 174). For the main dose, 10 ml of local anaesthetic will on average block the spinal nerves from C3 to T8. The more concentrated local anaesthetics may cause motor blockade of C2, C3 and C4, with paralysis of the diaphragm. Thus the less potent concentrations (1-1.5% lidocaine, 0.5% bupivacaine) are indicated.

Complications
See p. 175.
With this block there is always the danger of direct trauma to the spinal cord leading to neurological deficit in the trunk and limbs (upper and lower).

Thoracic epidural block

Lumbar epidural block is the most commonly used epidural technique because it is relatively easy and the needle is inserted below the termination of the spinal cord. Its disadvantage is that considerable volumes of solution have to be injected to reach the mid or upper thoracic nerves. Moreover there is inevitably blockade of the lumbar and sacral nerves. During abdominal operations, this is of little importance, but if the blockade is to be prolonged into the postoperative period for pain relief then the paralysis of the legs and perineum, together with the loss of sacral autonomic function (micturition, control of sphincters, etc.), presents problems for both patients and nursing staff.

If the epidural catheter can be placed at a point in the middle of the required band of analgesia, then much less drug can be used and unnecessary blockade of other nerves is prevented. The abdomen is supplied by the thoracic segments T6 to T12 (Fig. 161:1). To be at the centre of the required band of analgesia, the spinal canal must be entered through the thoracic intervertebral spaces, T10-T11 or T11-T12 for lower abdominal operations and T7-T8 or T8-T9 for upper abdominal operations. Even higher blocks can be used for thoracic operations to provide postoperative pain relief. Thoracic epidurals are also used for relieving the pain due to multiple fractured ribs.

Anatomy

The spinous processes of the thoracic vertebrae vary considerably in their angulation. The 1st, 2nd, 10th, 11th and 12th are, like the lumbar vertebrae, almost horizontal in the sagittal plane and allow a needle to be inserted at or near 90° to the skin. The other thoracic spinous processes are angled downwards to a greater or lesser extent and this requires a different technique to ensure entrance into the epidural space (Figs. 179:1 and 179:2).

Technical considerations

Entering the epidural space between T10-T11, T11-T12 or T12-L1 can be performed exactly as for lumbar epidural block. Because the spinous processes of T10, T11 and T12 are shorter than those of the lumbar vertebrae, the spinal canal is at a lesser depth from the skin. The needle should be inserted at right angles. The loss of resistance, as the ligamentum flavum is penetrated, will be easily determined.

It might be thought that it would be relatively easy to direct the catheter upwards and advance it to a higher level in the epidural space. However, this is unpredictable and the tip of the catheter may double back on itself. Thus if a high blockade is required it is best to insert the needle at the appropriate interspace.

Patient position

Lateral with spine fully flexed (knees raised in front of abdomen).

Landmarks

The spinous processes may be identified by their relationship to the iliac crest, the 12th rib and the scapula (Fig. 179:3). The most prominent process in the neck is C7.

Needle insertion

A skin wheal is raised with local anaesthetic over the chosen intervertebral space.

Fig. 179:1.
1. Inferior angle of scapulae (T7)
2. Rib margin 10 cm from midline (L2)
3. Superior aspect of iliac crest (L4)
4. Posterior superior iliac spine (S3)

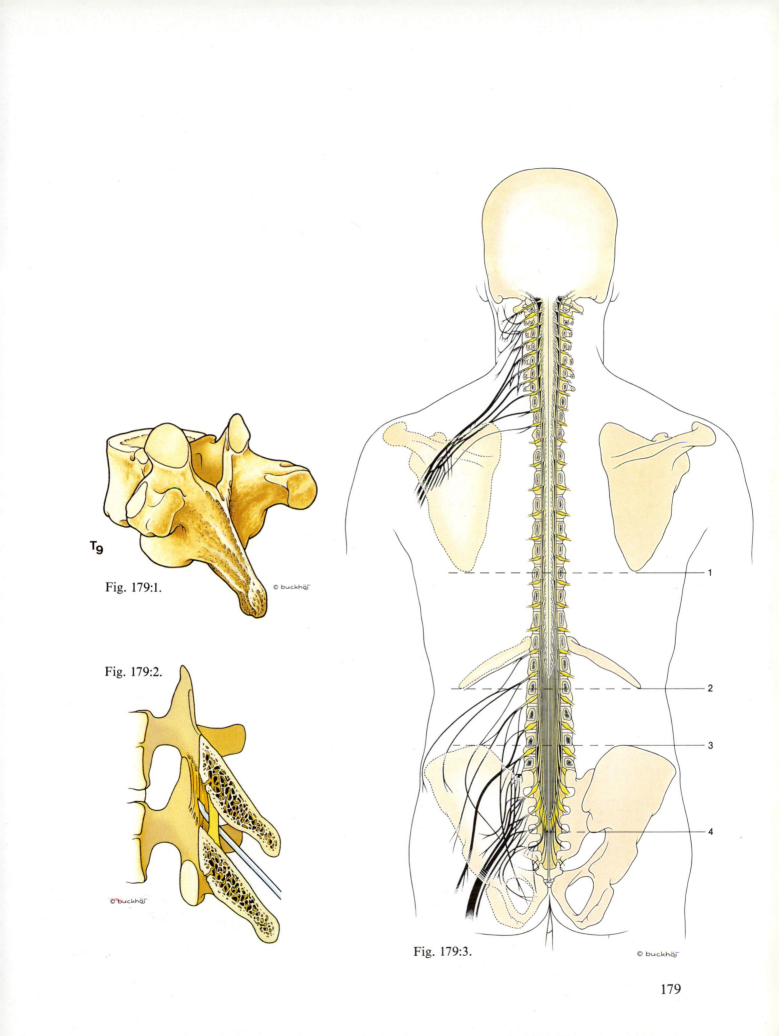

T₉

Fig. 179:1.

Fig. 179:2.

Fig. 179:3.

1

2

3

4

179

Midline approach

A needle inserted between the spinous processes in the midline has to be directed at an angle of about 45° to the skin so as to pass parallel to the spinous processes above and below (Figs. 181:1 and 181:2). The area of the ligamentum flavum accessible at this angle is rather less than with the right-angled approach lower down the spine. If bone is contacted and prevents the onward movement, then the anaesthetist must manipulate the needle so that it misses bone and continues on into the spinal canal. In most instances this can be accomplished without difficulty. Experience with a considerable number of lumbar epidural blocks is an advantage provided the more superficial position of the spinal canal is appreciated.

Paramedian or lateral approach

In the midthoracic region not only are the spinous processes very angulated, but also the laminae tend to overlap each other. Thus the paramedian approach, though avoiding the spinous processes, has to be at a relatively acute angle to negotiate the space between the laminae, which, of course, is occupied by the ligamentum flavum. The needle is inserted 1-1.5 cm from the upper border of the spinous process below the chosen interspace at an even more acute angle than in the midline approach. It is aimed medially but should avoid contact with the spinous processes (Fig. 181:3). If bone is contacted, it will therefore be the lamina, and the needle must be redirected to negotiate the space between the laminae.

The anaesthetist should have a good three-dimensional sense of the vertebral anatomy, and inspection of a skeleton helps considerably.

Because of the angulation of the needle, either with the midline or the lateral approach, the epidural space is entered at an acute angle with the curved end of the Tuohy needle nearest the dura (Fig. 181:4). Puncture of the dura is therefore less likely than with the horizontal approach in the lower thoracic or lumbar areas. Moreover the insertion of the catheter is easy and it will move cephalad without obstruction.

Catheter technique

See p. 172.

Drugs and dose

A test dose may be given (see p. 174). The main doses are given in Table 180:1.

Table 180:1.
Volumes used for thoracic epidural blockade

Indication	Volume (ml)
Upper abdominal surgery	10-15
Thoracic surgery	10-15
Postoperative pain relief	5-8

Complications

See p. 175.

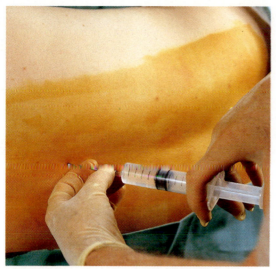

Fig. 181:1.

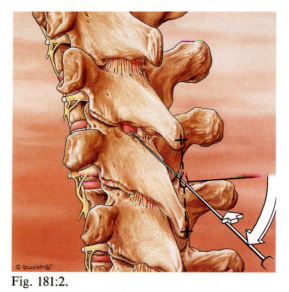

Fig. 181:2.

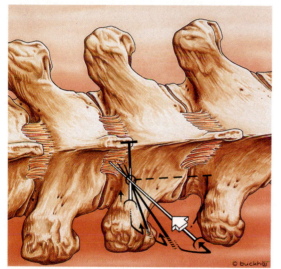

Fig. 181:3.

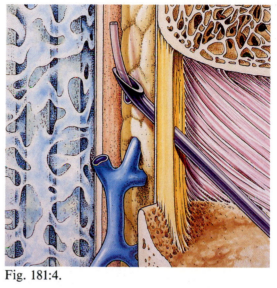

Fig. 181:4.

181

Caudal block

Theoretically caudal block can be used for any indication recommended for lumbar epidural block. However, there is often difficulty in getting the local anaesthetic to spread high enough. As a result the technique is generally reserved for procedures which require block-ade of the sacral nerves, though the lumbar and lower thoracic nerves can usually be block-ed with the appropriate dosage. Thus the main indications are:

1. Perineal operations
2. Inguinal and femoral herniorrhaphy
3. Cystoscopy and urethral surgery

Caudal block was widely used for relief of pain in labour but has largely been replaced by lumbar epidural block.

Anatomy

The sacrum is formed by the fusion of the five sacral vertebrae inside which the spinal canal continues its downward progress to end at the sacral hiatus, which is a gap in the fifth sacral vertebra due to the absence of its laminae (Fig. 183:1).

Occasionally the laminae of S4 and even S3 are also absent, causing an abnormally large hiatus. The sacral hiatus is covered by the sacro-coccygeal ligaments, which connect the coccyx to the sacrum (Fig. 183:2).

It is through this hiatus that the spinal canal may be entered when performing a caudal (sacral) block.

As the spinal cord ends at the level of L1-2, the lower lumbar and sacral nerve roots have a long course within the spinal canal, where they form the cauda equina (Fig. 183:3). The nerves are located initially in the subarachnoid space, and then leave at the termination of the dura mater at S1 to enter the sacral epidural space. The dorsal root ganglia of the sacral nerves may be grouped around the tip of the dural sac or may be some inches from it, near the inter-vertebral foramina.

Although it is usual for the spinal cord to end at L1-L2 and the dura mater at S2, varia-tions do occur and these may be of clinical im-portance if they are lower than normal.

Fig. 183:1. Courtesy of Astra.

Fig. 183:3.
1. *Cauda equina*
2. *Subarachnoid space*
3. *Dorsal root ganglion*
4. *Sacral epidural space*

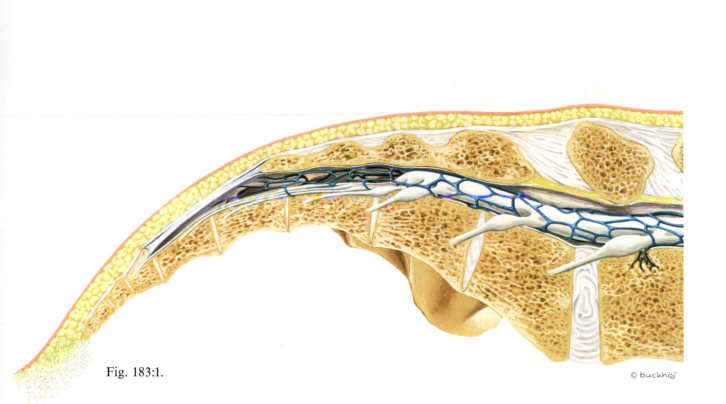

Fig. 183:1.

© buckhöj

Fig. 183:2.

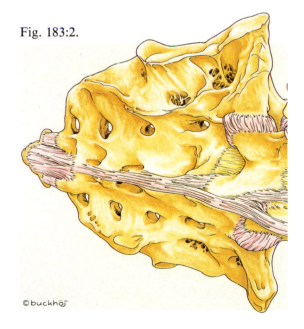

© buckhöj

Fig. 183:3.

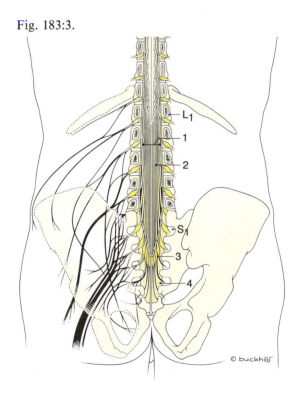

L₁

1

2

S₁

3

4

© buckhöj

Patient position

The patient may be placed laterally, or prone with a pillow under the pubis.

Landmarks

The sacral hiatus is palpated using the sacral cornua as the landmarks (Fig. 185:1).

Needle insertion

The skin is cleaned and the patient draped as for lumbar epidural block. An intradermal wheal is raised with local anaesthetic over the sacral hiatus (Fig. 185:2).

A needle is then inserted at 45° to the sacro-coccygeal ligament, which is pierced and the anterior wall of the sacral canal contacted (Fig. 185:3). The needle may then be redirected so that it is more in line with the sacral spinal canal (Fig. 185:5), and advanced 1-2 mm into the canal.

Various needles are available for caudal block, but a simple 4-cm, 21-23 gauge disposable needle is all that is required. If a catheter is being used, the needle must of course be of sufficiently large bore (16-18 gauge) to allow the catheter to pass through its lumen.

Injection of local anaesthetic is then made, observing the skin over the sacrum (Fig. 185:4). Should subcutaneous swelling occur, this would indicate a wrongly placed injection.

A finger palpating the sacro-coccygeal ligament during the initial injection will feel the ligament bulging outwards, thus confirming accurate placement.

Drugs and dose

A test dose (see p. 174) can be used.

Because the injection is made at one end of the epidural space rather than near the middle, it is more difficult to achieve spread into the thoracic region. Thus higher volumes of local anaesthetic are required than with lumbar epidural block. See Table 184:1 for adult dosage.

The most concentrated solutions are required for surgery. See p. 21.

Table 184:1.
Volumes used for caudal block (adults)

Operation	Volume (ml)
Lower abdominal	20-30
Lower limb & perineal	15-20

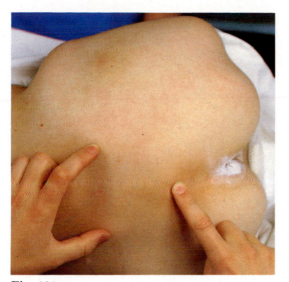

Fig. 185:1.

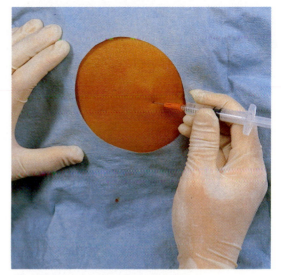

Fig. 185:2.

Fig. 185:3.

Fig. 185:4.

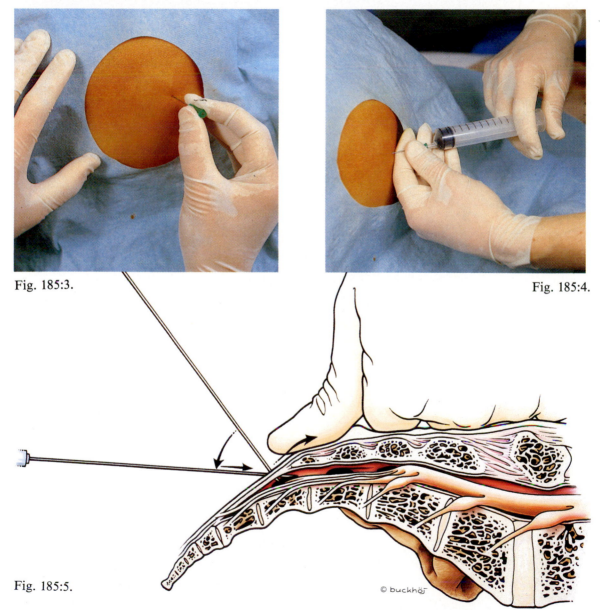

Fig. 185:5.

© buckhöj

185

Caudal block in paediatric surgery

Caudal block is quite easy to perform in children and has achieved popularity in operations such as herniorrhaphy and circumcision. It is usual to give the patient a light general anaesthetic before carrying out the block.

Dosage in children

In the literature there are widely differing recommendations given for the dosage of local anaesthetic to be used for caudal block in children. Most of the operations performed require nerve blocks to the height of T10.

It takes relatively small doses of local anaesthetic to achieve this level of block. Greater amounts will cause much higher blocks, but the disadvantage of this will not be apparent because children respond much less to widespread sympathetic blockade than do adults. In addition high systemic concentrations of local anaesthetics will not produce overt toxicity due to the concomitant use of general anaesthesia in these children. Thus considerable variations in dosage will have little effect upon the end result. Nevertheless, the use of excessive doses should be avoided. The recommendations given below have been set towards the lower end of the doses to be found in the literature.

There are two ways of calculating the dose, one based on body weight and the other on age. In normal sized children, either method can be used successfully, even though the relationship between age and weight is not linear. However, if the child is obese then there is a danger of overdosage and it is better to use age rather than body weight. Conversely, if the patient is obviously bigger or smaller than the average for his/her age, then the body weight should be used.

The two drugs most commonly used are lidocaine 1% and bupivacaine 0.25%. The choice lies in the desired duration of effect. The doses given below are therefore in millilitres and are the same for both drugs.

Age (yrs)	Dose (ml) for block to T12	Dose (ml) for block to T7
2	4	6
3	5	7.5
4	5.5	8
5	6	9
6	7	10.5
7	8	12
8	9	13.5
9	10	15
10	11	16.5

Body weight (kg)	Dose (ml) for block to T12	Dose (ml) for block to T7
10	3	4.5
12.5	4	6
15	5	7.5
17.5	6	9
20	7	10.5
22.5	8	12
25	9	13.5
27.5	10	15
30	11	16.5

Complications

See p. 175.

Suggested further reading

Bromage, P.R. (1978). Epidural Analgesia. W.B. Saunders, Philadelphia.

Covino, B.G. and Scott, D.B. (1985). Handbook of Epidural anaesthesia and analgesia. Schultz, Copenhagen.

Lee, J.A., Atkinson, R.S. and Watt, M.J. (1985). Sir Robert Macintosh's Lumbar punture and spinal analgesia. Churchill Livingstone, Edinburgh.

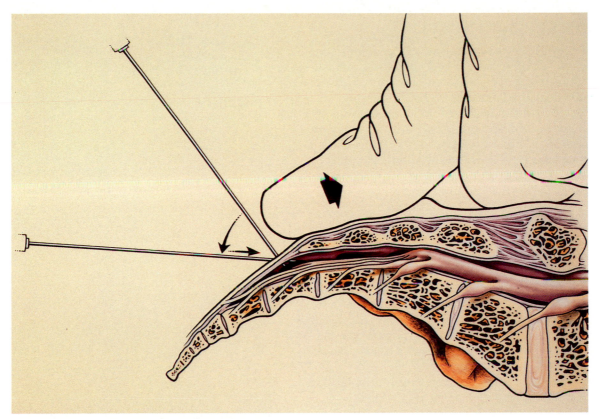

Fig. 187:1.

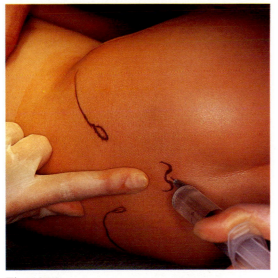

Fig. 187:2.

Spinal anaesthesia

Spinal anaesthesia is one of the oldest and most valuable of the techniques of regional anaesthesia. It is the most efficient of blocks, in that a small quantity of local anaesthetic injected into the spinal subarachnoid space will cause a widespread blockade of the spinal nerves. Systemic toxicity is therefore never a problem. However, though simple to perform, it does require a degree of understanding and training if it is to be used safely.

Anatomy

The spinal subarachnoid space communicates superiorly with the pontine cistern and the cerebello-medullary cistern (Fig. 189:1). It is situated between the pia and arachnoid maters and contains the cerebrospinal fluid (CSF), the spinal cord, the spinal nerves and the blood vessels supplying these structures. The arachnoid is closely applied, but not attached, to the dura mater.

The subarachnoid space ends at the level of the second sacral vertebra (Fig. 189:3).

The CSF is produced in the cerebral ventricles by the choroid plexuses. It circulates through the ventricular system and into the cerebral and spinal subarachnoid space. It is absorbed back into the blood through the arachnoid villi (Fig. 189:2) in the superior sagittal sinus and some of the other venous sinuses. The CSF in the spinal canal has little or no active circulation and drugs injected into it will spread mainly by diffusion before being absorbed into capillaries in the pia mater, the spinal nerves and the spinal cord.

Fig. 189:1 and 189:2.
1. *Arachnoid granulation*
2. *Dura mater (outer layer)*
3. *Dura mater (inner layer)*
4. *Subdural space*
5. *Arachnoid mater*
6. *Subarachnoid space*
7. *Superior sagittal sinus*
8. *Pia mater*
9. *Choroid plexus of 3rd ventricle*
10. *Great cerebral vein*
11. *Cisterna cerebellomedullaris*
12. *Interventricular foramen*
13. *Interpeduncular cistern*
14. *Cistern of the great cerebral vein (cisterna ambiens)*
15. *Choroid plexus of 4th ventricle*
16. *Foramen of Magendie*
17. *Superficial cerebral vein*
18. *Cerebral cortex*

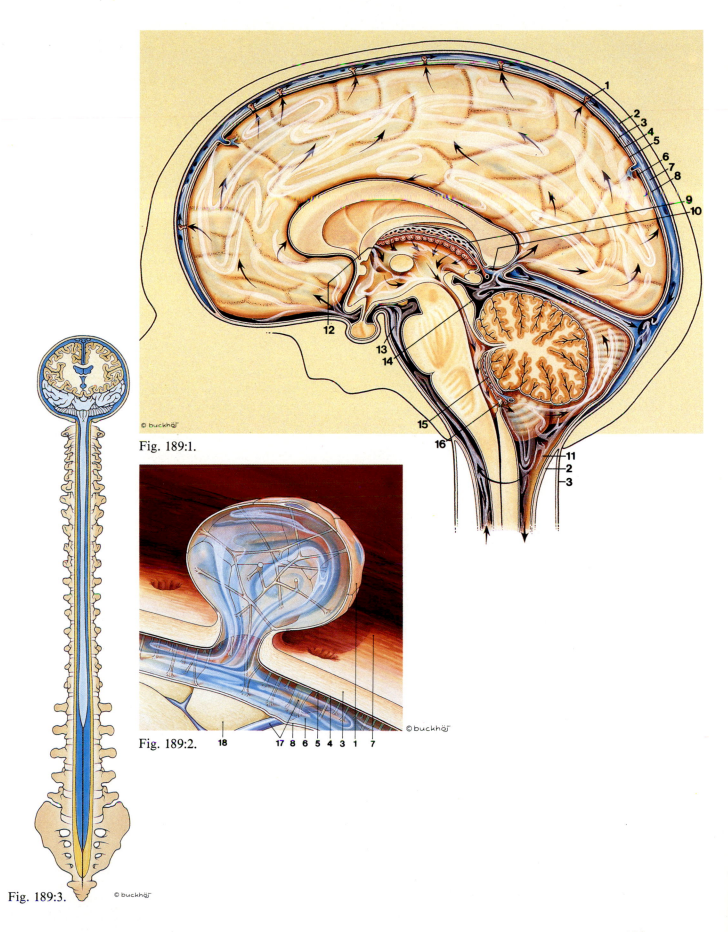

Fig. 189:1.

Fig. 189:2.

Fig. 189:3.

© buckhöj

Spinal nerves supply specific dermatomes in the body and different upper levels of block are required for different operations as follows:

Upper abdominal	T5 - 6
Lower abdominal	T8 - 9
Lower limb	T12
Perineal	S1
Bladder	T10
Kidney	T8

The spinal subarachnoid space is usually entered in the lumbar region (lumbar puncture), i.e. below the tip of the spinal cord. To reach the space, the needle must traverse the skin and subcutaneous tissue, the supraspinous ligament, the intraspinous ligament, the ligamentum flavum, the dura mater and the arachnoid mater.

Equipment
Spinal anaesthesia should always be carried out with full aseptic and antiseptic precautions.

Spinal needles
Spinal needles are supplied with stylets and the most commonly used vary from 22-26 French gauge. The smaller the bore of the needle, the less risk there is of post-lumbar puncture headache. Only the 22 gauge can be inserted reliably without the aid of an introducer. Thinner needles bend too easily and most of the penetration of the ligaments must be done with a short stout introducer through which the spinal needle can be inserted before the final penetration into the subarachnoid space. Disposable needles are available and a 25 gauge will easily pass through a short (4-cm) 18 gauge hypodermic needle.

Spinal pack
The spinal pack should also include:

1. Sterile drapes
2. Lotion bowel for antiseptic
3. 2-ml and 5-ml syringes
4. Needle for aspirating local anaesthetic from its ampoule
5. Ampoule of local anaesthetic. Though some drugs can be autoclaved repeatedly, it is better that this is only done once. Ampoules in sterile packages are also available and can be "dropped" aseptically onto the sterile trolley. In drawing up solution from an ampoule, care must be taken to avoid glass fragments entering the syringe. This can be done by not "grounding" the aspiration needle on the bottom of the ampoule, or by using a filter.
6. Swabs

Patient position
1. Lateral with the spine maximally flexed by raising the knees and flexing the neck and thorax.

2. Sitting with spine maximally flexed by resting the feet on a stool and bending the trunk forward towards thighs.

If flexion is limited, either the paramedian (lateral) approach to the lumbar interspaces or a lumbosacral approach may be used.

Landmarks
Lumbar spinous processes. The iliac crest is at the level of the fourth lumbar vertebra.

Drugs and dose

Virtually all local anaesthetics can and have been used for spinal anaesthesia. They may be divided into:

1. Short acting (1-1½h):
   lidocaine, mepivacaine, procaine *2cc min*
2. Medium/long acting (1½-4 h):
   tetracaine, bupivacaine, cinchocaine

Duration is considerably affected by dosage.

Drugs used for spinal anaesthesia are also categorised by their specific gravity (S.G.) in relation to that of the CSF, which is around 1.003 at 37°C.

There is considerable confusion regarding specific gravities because these change considerably in the temperature range from 18-37°C. Thus a solution which is hyperbaric at room temperature may become hypobaric when it has warmed to body temperature. In practice there seems to be little difference in the behaviour of so-called isobaric and hypobaric solutions, both of which are largely unaffected by gravity, i.e. by the patient's posture during and after injection. Hypobaric solutions are perforce of low concentration and have often to be used in larger volumes. They will therefore take longer to reach 37°C and during this time they will be iso- or hyperbaric. It is not possible to make solutions markedly "lighter" than CSF but it is easy to make them much heavier.

Hyperbaric solutions are made by the addition of glucose 5-9%, giving an S.G. of 1.020-1.030. They are affected by gravity after injection and are also less miscible with CSF. In patients kept horizontal throughout, they tend to spread more cephalad than isobaric solutions.

The most commonly employed drugs are:

Lidocaine
Available as a 5% solution in 7.5% glucose (hyperbaric). Dose 1-3 ml. Also effective as a 2% plain solution (isobaric), in a dose of 3-6 ml.

Mepivacaine
Available as 4% solution in 9.5% glucose (hyperbaric). Dose 1-3 ml. Also effective as a 2% plain solution (isobaric), in a dose of 3-6 ml.

Procaine
Usually supplied in solid crystalline form which dissolves in CSF. Procaine solutions over 2.5% concentration are hyperbaric. Dose 100-200 mg.

Tetracaine
This is available as a 1% solution which may be diluted to 0.5% with 10% glucose (hyperbaric), normal saline (hypobaric) or water (isobaric). It is also supplied as a crystalline powder which may be dissolved in CSF. The dose is 1-4 ml (5-20 mg of the powder).

Bupivacaine
Available as 0.5% in 8% glucose (hyperbaric) or as the plain 0.5% solution (isobaric). Dose 2-4 ml. In the USA 0.75% in 8.25% glucose is available (hypobaric). Dose 1-2 ml.

Cinchocaine (Dibucaine)
Available as 0.5% in 6% glucose (hyperbaric). Dose 2-3 ml. Also supplied as a hypobaric solution, 0.067% in buffered saline, dose 5-10 ml.

Needle insertion

Midline approach

Having identified the appropriate intervertebral space, the skin is held firmly against the
adjacent spinous process while the needle or
introducer is directed in a slightly cephalad direction in the midline, so as to pass equidistant
between the spinous processes. The bevel
should be pointing laterally (Fig. 193:1). No infiltration of the skin is necessary if a fine needle or a sharp introducer is used. The increased
resistance of the ligamentum flavum is often
felt. When it is thought that the spinal canal
has been entered, the stylet is withdrawn and
the needle hub examined for CSF leakage.

If an introducer is used, it should only be inserted as far as the ligamentum flavum, i.e.
when it is firmly engaged in the ligaments.
Even a short introducer can reach and pierce
the dura mater in some patients, increasing the
risk of headache. Once firmly held by the ligaments, the fine spinal needle is pushed through
it and on into the spinal canal (Figs. 193:2 and
193:3). Withdrawal of the stylet will reveal the
escape of CSF. CSF leakage can be rather slow
with 25 and 26 gauge needles. Ideally CSF
should continue to escape while the needle
bevel is rotated slowly through 360° (Fig.
193:4).

Should bone be contacted relatively superficially, it is probably the lamina of the vertebra.
The needle or introducer must be withdrawn
almost back to the skin and redirected (usually
more cephalad). Because of their lack of rigid-
ity it is not possible to redirect fine needles
once they are engaged in ligament.
   If bone is contacted deeply, it may be the anterior wall of the spinal canal. The stylet
should be withdrawn and the needle retracted
slowly while observing any leakage of CSF at
the needle hub.

Fig. 193:4. Courtesy of Astra.

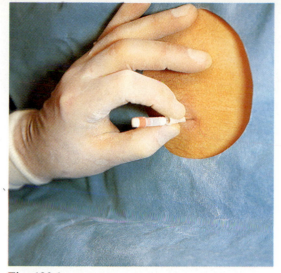

Fig. 193:1.

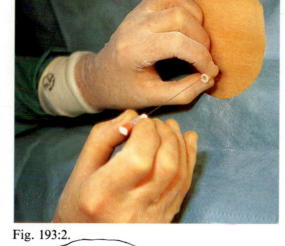

Fig. 193:2.

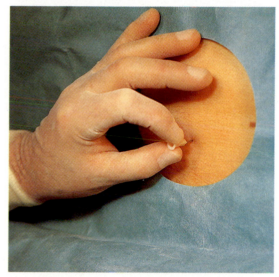

Fig. 193:3.

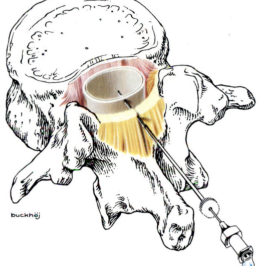

Fig. 193:4.

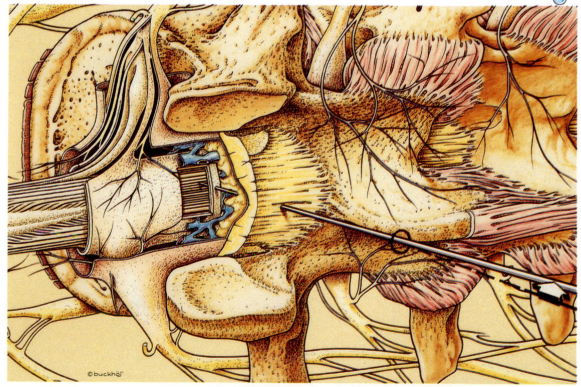

Fig. 193:5.

Paramedian or lateral approach

The needle or introducer is inserted 2 cm lateral to the spinous process below the selected interspace. It is directed upwards and medially. If bone is contacted it is probably the inferior surface of the lamina above the space, and the needle should be redirected more caudally (Figs. 195:1 and 195:2).

Lumbosacral (Taylor) approach

The needle is inserted 1 cm medial and 1 cm caudad to the posterior superior iliac spine. It is directed medially and cephalad, and roughly parallel to the dorsal surface of the sacrum (Figs. 195:3 and 195:4). The needle tip should reach the lumbosacral interspace in the midline. If bone is contacted it is probably the posterior surface of the sacrum and the needle must be directed more cephalad.

Injection of local anaesthetic

There is no point in injecting local anaesthetic if the needle tip is not unequivocally within the subarachnoid space, as shown by CSF leakage or easy aspiration of CSF with a syringe.

A syringe containing the calculated dose is attached to the needle hub and the plunger withdrawn a small distance to confirm the aspiration of CSF. The needle hub must be firmly held by the non-dominant hand during attachment of the syringe, aspiration and injection. Even a small movement may cause displacement of the needle tip.

A simple straightforward injection is all that is required. Barbotage is not feasible with small gauge needles and is unnecessary. Using a 5-ml syringe and a hyperbaric solution with dextrose, 1 ml every 5 s is the maximum rate of injection that can be made.

The needle is withdrawn and the patient turned into the desired position.

Continuous spinal anaesthesia

As with epidural blockade, spinal anaesthesia may be prolonged by using a catheter technique. To insert a standard epidural catheter into the subarachnoid space, a size 18 gauge Tuohy needle is required and a large hole will be made in the dura mater. The risk of headache is therefore much higher then when using a fine bore needle. However, if the technique is used with elderly patients, the incidence of post-spinal headache is remarkably low and it is in the elderly that the main advantages over epidural block are evident. These include the reliable reproduction of a block with a top-up injection, the use of very small amounts of local anaesthetic drug and the ability to easily modify the height of the block knowing the response to the initial injection.

A catheter for use with a 22 gauge needle is available. Very small bore catheters capable of being inserted through 25 or 26 gauge needles are available for industrial use and could have a place in this type of block.

If continuous spinal blockade is used, the aseptic precautions, particularly the use of a bacterial filter at the catheter end, must be rigorously followed.

Combined spinal and epidural block

Some authorities like first to insert an epidural needle into the epidural space. A fine bore needle can then be passed through it into the subarachnoid space. After injecting local anaesthetic, the spinal needle is withdrawn and a catheter passed into the epidural space. In this way the advantage of a rapid onset spinal block can be combined with which may be prolonged epidural block.

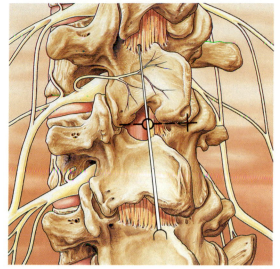

Fig. 195:1.

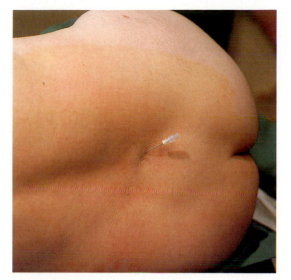

Fig. 195:2.

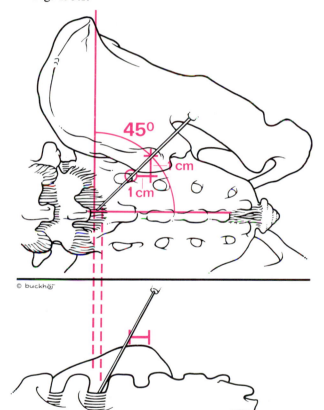

45⁰

cm

1 cm

© buckhöj

Fig. 195:3.

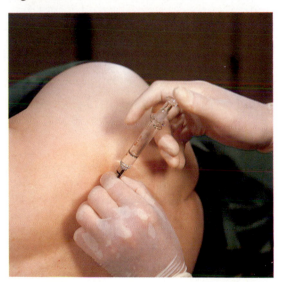

Fig. 195:4.

Factors affecting the spread of spinal anaesthesia

The number of spinal nerves that will be blocked following an intrathecal injection of local anaesthetic depends on many factors such as the dose and baricity of the solution, and the posture of the patient. Though it is often believed that spinal anaesthesia is very predictable and easy to manipulate in regard to the height of block, Bier described it as "capricious", which it certainly is. Thus in spite of the best endeavours of the anaesthetist, considerable variations can and do occur and must be reckoned with.

1. Dosage would appear an obvious factor; increasing it would surely increase the spread. However, it has become clear that the relationship between dose and spread is not linear. Studies have shown only a minor additional spread when the dose of 0.5% hyperbaric bupivacaine is increased from 3 to 5 ml. In the range of 1-3 ml there are differences in the height of blockade, especially if the patient is sitting up for a few minutes after the injection, i.e. gravity is also affecting the spread.

2. Gravity can influence the height of spread but less than might be imagined, and only with hyperbaric solutions. Iso- and hypobaric solutions are virtually unaffected by posture as they mix easily and rapidly with CSF. Gravity only causes major differences in spread when it is maximal, i.e. when the patient's spine is vertical. Thus a small quantity, 1-1.5 ml, of hyperbaric solution will give a block confined to the sacral roots (a saddle block) if the patient is kept sitting up during and for several minutes after the injection. Using a larger volume, 3-4 ml, the difference between sitting up and lying down becomes much less marked.

Unilateral block can be obtained as long as the patient is kept in the lateral position. However, once the supine position is resumed, the block rapidly becomes bilateral.

The head-down position which should enhance cephalad spread, only increases the height of block to a small extent.

Changing posture involves movement of the spine and some authorities believe that this, and the associated movement of the spinal cord and spinal nerves within the subarachnoid space, can enhance the spread. Turning from a lateral position to the opposite lateral position has been claimed to considerably increase the height of block in patients undergoing Caesarean section.

3. Baricity. Even in the horizontal position, hyperbaric solutions in doses up to 3 ml produce higher blocks than isobaric or plain solutions. It may well be that the relative non-miscibility of glucose-containing solutions together with their hyperbaricity allows them to ascend into the thoracic part of the subarachnoid space, with gravity assisting the movement of drug in the natural curves of the spine.

4. Late pregnancy. Though a satisfactory direct comparison of spinal anaesthesia in late pregnancy and in the non-pregnant state is difficult if not impossible, there is clinical evidence to suggest that spinal blockade achieves higher levels in late pregnancy than at other times, and very high blocks may be encountered.

Factors affecting duration of spinal anaesthesia

1. Drug and dosage. The obvious way to control the duration of spinal block is to use a local anaesthetic with appropriate duration of effect. However, there is good evidence that duration is also closely related to dosage, the higher doses causing longer blocks than the lower.

2. Vasoconstrictors such as epinephrine or phenylephrine have been shown to prolong spinal blockade, though there are differences in opinion regarding the clinical usefulness of this. The actual mode of action of vasoconstrictors within the subarachnoid space has not been defined, though it is clearly not identical with their mode of action at other sites.

There appears to be a difference in the prolongation according to the local anaesthetic drug used, the best effect being with tetracaine and the least with lidocaine and bupivacaine.

Vasoconstrictors appear to be able to cause very prolonged block (>8 h) in some patients, but their action is unpredictable in an individual.

If used, the recommended dosage is epinephrine 0.1 mg (0.1 ml of 1:1.000 solution) or phenylephrine 1 mg.

Failure of spinal blockade

This may be a partial failure, i.e. inability to reach a sufficiently high blockade, or a total failure in which little or no nerve block is apparent after 15-20 min.

Partial failure may be due to inadequate dosage but is more likely due to the wide individual variations that occur with spinal anaesthesia.

Total failure to produce a demonstrable nerve block does occur and will raise the issue of whether the local anaesthetic drug has deteriorated in the ampoule or there has been a problem during the sterilising process. Neither of these possibilities is very likely however. Given that local anaesthetic in adequate dose injected into the CSF **must** produce multiple spinal nerve block, one is left with the inescapable conclusion that during the injection the needle tip was **not** in the subarachnoid space. This could be due to slight movement during the injection, or the bevel of the needle being only partially inserted through the dura etc.

Whether the failure is partial or total, the anaesthetist should have a pre-arranged contingency plan. If the block has "missed" one or two dermatomes, this might be made good with a subcutaneous infiltration at the incision or the IV injection of a short acting opioid. If the failure is total, then there may have to be recourse to a general anaesthesia. Each patient will present an individual problem with a variety of solutions.

Complications
Hypotension
Widespread sympathetic blockade can cause a reduction in peripheral resistance due to vasodilatation. Because the venous capacitance is also increased, any impediment to venous return (e.g. head-up posture or caval occlusion) will cause a fall in cardiac output.

Hypotension may also be contributed to by hypovolaemia or caval occlusion, both of which require a degree of vasoconstriction to maintain a normal arterial pressure.

Sudden severe hypotension during spinal block in a conscious patient is usually due to vaso-vagal fainting. This is accompanied by pallor, bradycardia, nausea and vomiting and sweating. Patients may suffer a transient vagal cardiac arrest and can develop signs of coronary insufficiency. Consciousness will be lost during this period of arrest. This type of hypotension is not seen in patients given a concomitant general anaesthetic. Although a general anaesthetic enhances the hypotensive effects of a spinal block, the decrease in arterial pressure is not precipitate and not accompanied by vagal activity with a marked bradycardia.

Treatment
If posture or caval occlusion are thought to be factors, the patient should be repostured without delay, e.g. left lateral and head down.

Because vasodilatation is the trigger to most hypotensive episodes, it is logical to give a vasopressor (see p. 24) which will usually act rapidly and effectively. Overdosage causing **hyper**tension is to be avoided. In late pregnancy the effect of vasopressors on uterine blood flow is often feared, but an adverse effect on the foetus is unlikely if overshoot hypertension is avoided, whereas prolonged hypotension will be deleterious to the foetus.

Fluids are of use if there is evidence of hypovolaemia, but they should be backed up with vasopressors if the arterial pressure is not rapidly restored.

Atropine may be used for severe bradycardia, but vasopressors with both α- and β-receptor activity, e.g. ephedrine, will increase the heart rate satisfactorily by themselves.

Total spinal anaesthesia
If by accident an excessive amount of local anaesthetic is injected into the subarachnoid space a high or total spinal anaesthetic will ensue. This will involve widespread paralysis with respiratory arrest, severe hypotension and, if there is substantial cranial spread, unconsciousness. All these will appear within a few minutes of the injection.

Treatment is by artificial ventilation and vasopressor support of the circulation. Though alarming, total spinal block can be effectively treated if the diagnosis is made promptly.

Neurological damage
See p. 25.

Headache
See p. 176.

Thoracic spinal block

This technique is mainly used for the relief of cancer pain involving one or more thoracic spinal nerves. The object is to block only the appropriate nerves unilaterally and not to cause a widespread block, particularly if neurolytic agents such as phenol or alcohol are being used.

Patient position

The lateral position is used so that the spine can be easily flexed (Fig. 199:1). Phenol solutions are hyperbaric and the side to be blocked should be underneath. If alcohol is used, it is hypobaric and the affected side should be uppermost. To be sure that the posterior roots of the spinal nerves are the most affected, it should be possible to gently roll the patients up to 45° backwards with phenol or 45° forward with alcohol after the needle insertion and before the injection is made.

It should be remembered that adopting the correct position may be very painful for some patients.

Needle insertion

It is best to use a 22 gauge needle rather than a 25 or 26 gauge as the escape of cerebrospinal fluid (CSF) is more quickly seen when the subarachnoid space is entered (Fig. 199:2).

The thoracic puncture is done either in the midline (Figs. 199:1 and 199:2) or laterally (Figs. 199:3 and 199:4) as with thoracic epidural block (see p. 178). As the needle advances, it will be felt to "click" through the ligamentum flavum. At this point, the stilette should be removed and the needle advanced a millimetre at a time, waiting to observe any escape of CSF. Once the dura is punctured, CSF will appear at the needle hub. The patient is then gently rolled forwards (for alcohol) or backwards (for phenol), ensuring the continuing escape of CSF.

Drugs and dose

Phenol 6-10% in glycerine or absolute alcohol. Injection is made using a Tuberculin (1 ml) syringe. Aliquots of 0.25 ml are used and after each injection, the patient is observed and questioned for paraesthesia and/or analgesia in the required spinal segments, allowing 3-5 min after each injection. Once the desired band of anaesthesia is obtained, the needle is withdrawn. The patient should remain immobile in the same position for 30 min.

Complications

1. Unwanted blockade of spinal segments outwit the painful area
2. Motor blockade leading to muscle weakness
3. Neuropathy of the spinal nerves
4. Urinary or faecal incontinence

The nerve block should last 2-3 months but may be much shorter, in which case it will have to be repeated.

Suggested further reading

Greene, N.M. (1981). The physiology of spinal anesthesia. Williams and Wilkins, Baltimore.

Greene N.M. (1985). Distribution of local anesthetic solutions within the subarachnoid space. Anesth. Analg. 64, 715.

Katz, J. and Renck, H. (1987). Handbook of Thoraco-abdominal Nerve Block. Mediglobe, Fribourg.

Lee, J.A., Atkinson, R.S. and Watt, M.J. (1985). Sir Robert Macintosh's Lumbar punture and spinal analgesia. Churchill Livingstone, Edinburgh.

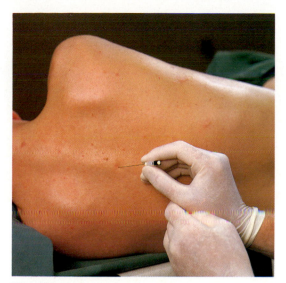

Fig. 199:1.

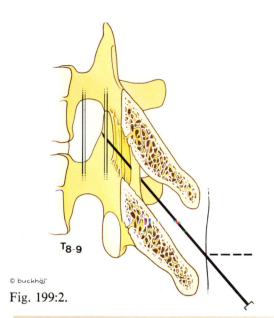

T8-9

© buckhöj

Fig. 199:2.

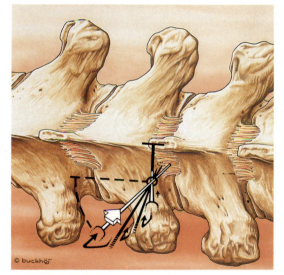

© buckhöj

Fig. 199:3.

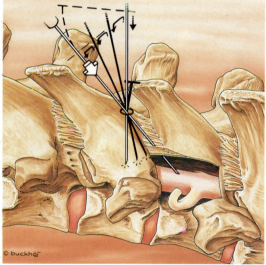

© buckhöj

Fig. 199:4.

Sympathetic nerve blockade

Anatomy

The sympathetic nervous system contains both afferent and efferent nerve fibres. They enter or leave the spinal cord in the 14 spinal nerves from T1 to L2, though some authorities believe that cervical nerves are also involved.

Efferent fibres leave the spinal nerves as they exit from the spinal canal, and run as white rami communicantes to reach the sympathetic chain. Here they may run up or down to reach a synapse in a ganglion from which emerges a post-synaptic fibre. These run back to the spinal nerves as grey rami communicantes and are distributed to their end organs in the distribution of the spinal nerve. Some efferent fibres do not synapse in the sympathetic chain but rather leave it to reach a synapse in a ganglion of the visceral plexuses, e.g. the coeliac, aortic or hypogastric.

Efferent fibres supply blood vessels, visceral organs, sweat glands and hair follicles.

Afferent fibres arise from the visceral organs and the blood vessels and pass through the sympathetic chain without synapsing to reach the dorsal horn of the spinal cord. Like somatic sensory fibres, their nerve cells lie within the dorsal nerve ganglia. Afferent fibres are responsible for visceral reflexes and visceral sensations such as nausea, hunger and bladder distension. They are also responsible for certain types of pain, e.g. colic, uterine contractions, and the pain of ischaemia, such as angina or the rest pain in ischaemic limbs. In certain disorders (reflex sympathetic dystrophies) they cause inappropriate pain such as causalgia.

Indications for sympathetic blockade

These include:

1. Peripheral vascular disease of the lower limbs. Sympathectomy relieves rest pain and improves the blood supply to the skin.

2. Visceral pain in conditions such as pancreatitis or cancer.

3. Causalgia.

4. Pain of herpes zoster.

5. Acute vasoconstrictions of arteries, e.g. with frostbite or arterial embolism.

Sympathetic blockade may be transient if local anaesthetics are used, or permanent (or semi-permanent) if neurolytic drugs such as phenol or alcohol are used. These agents are not suitable in certain areas, such as the stellate ganglia, and blockade must be performed with local anaesthetic drugs given frequently to try to break the vicious circle of inappropriate pain due to reflex dystrophy.

The sympathetic nerves can be blocked in the sympathetic chain, in the autonomic plexuses (stellate or coeliac), in the splanchnic nerves or in the epidural space. Because several of the blocks require deep penetration with the needle and accurate placement, radiological control, preferably with an image intensifier, is indispensable.

Fig. 203.1
1. Superior cervical ganglion
2. Middle cervical ganglion
3. Stellate ganglion
4. Coeliac ganglion
5. Superior mesenteric ganglion
6. Inferior mesenteric ganglion
7. Superior hypogastric plexus

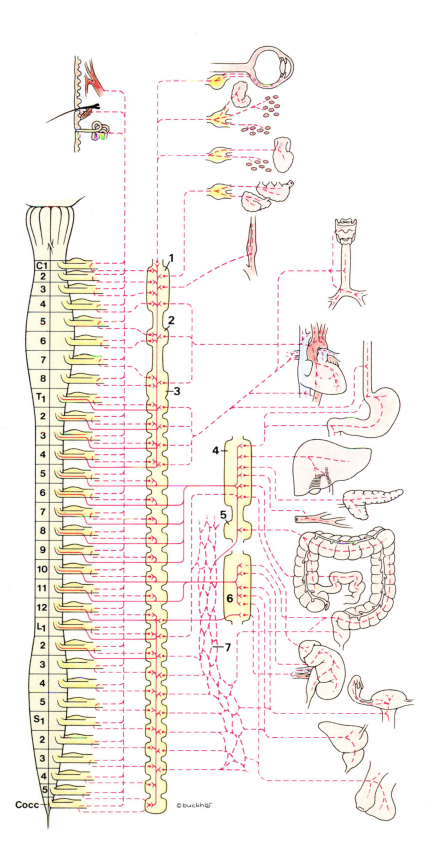

Fig. 203:1.

Lumbar sympathectomy

Anatomy
The sympathetic chain runs on the anterolateral aspect of the vertebral column (Figs. 205:1 and 2). In the lumbar region it lies on the medial margin of the psoas muscle, in the retroperitoneal space, behind the aorta on the left side and behind the inferior vena cava on the right.

Patient position
Lateral, with side to be blocked uppermost.

Landmarks
1. The midline
2. The 12th rib
3. The iliac crest

Needle insertion
A wheal is raised 8-10 cm lateral to the midline at the level of the midpoint between (2) and (3). A long (15-cm) needle is inserted and directed anteriorly and medially at 45° to the skin. The object is to contact the body of the third lumbar vertebra. Once the bone is felt, the needle is redirected less medially so as to glide past the lateral margin of the vertebral body. Using radiographic control, the needle tip is positioned so that it is just behind the anterior border of the vertebral body (lateral view) and medial to the lateral border (anteroposterior view). Aspiration or frank escape of blood from the needle hub indicates penetration into a blood vessel such as the aorta, the vena cava or a paravertebral vein.

Radio-opaque dye (1-2 ml) is injected using flexible plastic tubing while watching the X-ray screen. It should remain close to the anterolateral aspect of the vertebral body (Fig. 205:3).

Misplacement can be diagnosed as follows:
1. If the dye streaks laterally and inferiorly from the vertebra (Fig. 205:5), the needle tip is within the psoas muscle. It must be reinserted more medially.
2. If dye spreads markedly anterior to the vertebra, the needle tip is intraperitoneal.
3. If dye outlines the paravertebral veins, the tip is intravenous.
4. If dye is seen between adjacent vertebrae, it is within the substance of the intervertebral disc. That the needle tip was not lying between the vertebrae and therefore possibly within the disc should have been obvious before injecting the dye.

The fact that misplacement can so easily occur is the major argument for insisting on radiological control.

Drugs and dose
If a local anaesthetic is being used, 10 ml of 1% lidocaine or 0.25% bupivacaine or their equivalent (see p. 20). A longer block can be obtained with 0.5% bupivacaine. In selected cases a catheter can be used and repeated doses of local anaesthetic given.

For a permanent or semipermanent sympathetic block, 10 ml of 6-10% phenol may be used. This volume will spread over two to three vertebrae and only a single injection is necessary for each side to be blocked. Multiple needling is unnecessary. Radio-opaque dye should be added to confirm the correct placement and spread of the main dose.

Complications
1. Misplaced injection (intravascular, intrapsoas, intraspinal, etc.) should be ruled out by the X-ray confirmation of the needle position before injecting the phenol or local anaesthetic. X-ray control should be considered mandatory for this block because of the disastrous effects of a misplaced injection of phenol into, say, the subarachnoid space.

2. Intrapsoas injection (Fig. 205:5). An injection into the psoas muscle can still produce an adequate sympathectomy because it will block the postganglionic fibres which leave the sympathetic chain and run into the psoas muscle to reach the nerves of the lumbar plexus. However, it will not cause destruction of the sympathetic chain and is sometimes associated with neuropathy of one of the somatic nerves of the lumbar plexus. This will usually disappear eventually but can cause some weeks or months of discomfort.

Fig. 205:3 and 205:4
The dye should remain close to the anterolateral aspect of the vertebrae. A single injection (8 ml) will cover three to five vertebrae.
Courtesy of Dr. D.G. Littlewood.

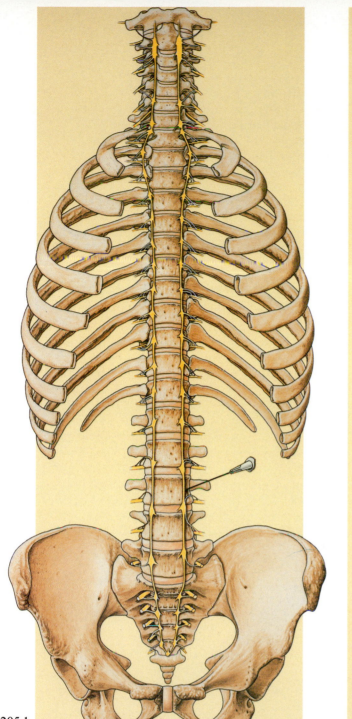

Fig. 205:1.

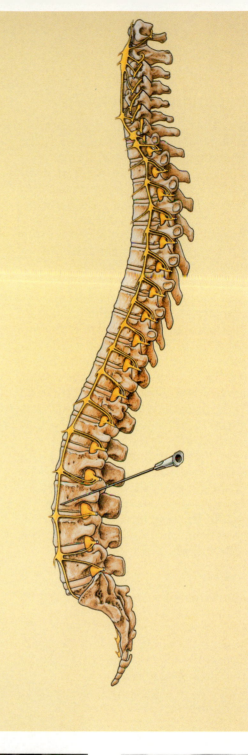

Fig. 205:2.

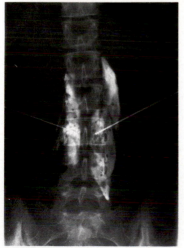

Fig. 205:3.

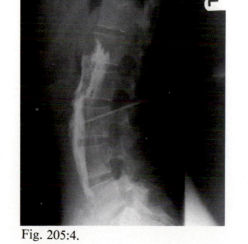

Fig. 205:4.

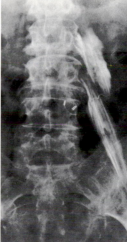

Fig. 205:5.

205

Stellate ganglion blockade

Anatomy

The stellate (cervico-thoracic) ganglion is the lowest of the three ganglia of the cervical sympathetic nervous system. The cervical sympathetic chain receives its preganglionic fibres from the upper thoracic nerves, there being no white rami communicantes from the cervical nerves. Thus all the central connections from the cervical sympathetic system must either pass through, or synapse in, the stellate ganglion.

The three ganglia and the sympathetic chain lie on the prevertebral fascia in the neck. The superior cervical ganglia is at the level of the second and third cervical vertebrae, the middle is at the level of the sixth vertebra and the stellate is at the level of the seventh vertebra between the base of the transverse process and the neck of the first rib.

The term "stellate ganglion blockade" is not strictly correct as the injection is made above the level of the ganglion and enough local anaesthetic is injected to spread up and down to anaesthetise all three ganglia, or, at the least, all the central connections of the cervical sympathetic system (Figs. 206:1 and 207:2).

Blockade of the cervical sympathetic system on one side leads to widespread effects including:

1. Dilatations of the blood vessels of the head, neck and upper limb. This can cause "stuffiness" in the ipsilateral nostril.

2. Absence of sweating in the same area.

3. Constriction of the pupil.

4. Ptosis of the upper eyelid.

The system also supplies many other structures, including the heart, the pharynx, the thyroid and the carotid body, but effects on these structures would only be evident with a bilateral block, which is not recommended.

(2), (3) and (4) above are components of Horner's syndrome, which appears with a successful stellate ganglion block.

Indications

Stellate ganglion block has been used for a wide variety of conditions, including:

1. Raynaud's phenomenon
2. Causalgia or other reflex sympathetic dystrophies in the upper limb
3. To relieve arterial vasoconstriction in the upper limb, e.g. following intra-arterial injection of thiopental, frostbite or following microsurgical operation
4. Herpes zoster
5. Hyperhidrosis

Because a single injection of local anaesthetic will only have a short-lived effect, it is necessary to reblock the stellate ganglion at frequent intervals to try to break the vicious circle causing the pain. A catheter technique similar to that of epidural block can be used for continuous blockade.

The use of neurolytics is generally inadvisable due to the proximity of the brachial plexus and the phrenic nerves, not to mention other important structures in the neck. Stellate ganglion block has been used as a predictor of effect prior to surgical excision of the ganglion, but this is a potentially very hazardous operation.

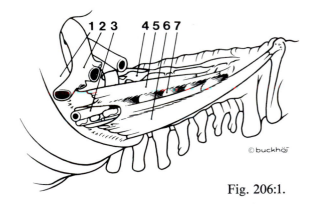

Fig. 206:1.

1. First rib
2. Subclavian vein
3. Subclavian artery
4. Stellate ganglion
5. Anterior scalene muscle
6. Middle scalene muscle
7. Transverse process of C6

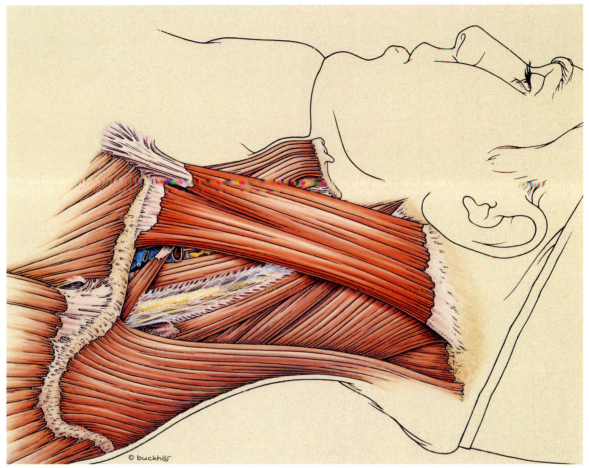

Fig. 207:1.

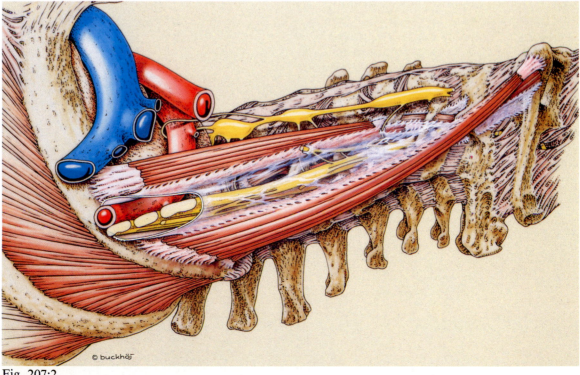

Fig. 207:2.

Patient position
Supine with head raised and extended, as for endotracheal intubation.

Landmarks
1. The cricoid cartilage (which is at the level of the 6th cervical vertebra) and the trachea
2. The sternomastoid muscle
3. The carotid artery
4. The transverse process of C6, felt by palpating between (2) and (3) laterally and (1) medially

Needle insertion
Using two fingers of the non-dominant hand to palpate the transverse process and to hold the skin immobile, a short (4-cm) 22 gauge needle is inserted between the trachea medially and the sternomastoid and carotid artery laterally (Fig. 209:1). It is directed perpendicularly backwards until it contacts bone (the transverse process of C6). If it meets resistance which is not clearly bony, it may be in contact with the interspinous ligament or the insertion of the longus colli muscle (Fig. 209:2). It should be withdrawn and reinserted until bone is felt. The needle is then withdrawn 1-2 mm and held firmly while an assistant attaches a flexible cannula and syringe (Figs. 209:3 and 209:4).

Drugs and dose
After careful aspiration, inject 10 ml of 1% lidocaine or 0.25% bupivacaine or their equivalent (see p. 20). More dilute solutions will be effective but will have a shorter duration. Larger doses (up to 20 ml) may be required to ensure sympathetic blockade to the arm.

A successful injection will be indicated by the rapid onset (within 5 min) of a Horner's syndrome and dilatation of the veins in the ipsilateral upper limb.

Complications
1. Blockade of the phrenic nerve or recurrent laryngeal nerves. These will usually cause only minor symptoms such as hoarseness and dysphagia, and are more common when larger volumes (20 ml) are used.

2. Intra-arterial injection into the vertebral artery can cause a major toxic reaction even with small quantities of local anaesthetic as all the injected drug goes immediately to the brain. Penetration of the arterial wall is, however, usually obvious by refluxed blood.

3. Intraspinal injection, either epidural or subarachnoid, can occur if the needle has entered an intervertebral foramen or the dural cuff of a cervical spinal nerve.

4. Haematoma in the neck.

Fig. 209:1.
1. *Cricoid cartilage*
2. *Stellate ganglion*
3. *Middle cervical ganglion*
4. *Transverse process of C6*

Fig. 209:3. Courtesy of Astra.
1. *Transverse process of C6*
2. *Vertebral artery*
3. *Sternomastoid muscle*
4. *Common carotid artery*
5. *Stellate ganglion*

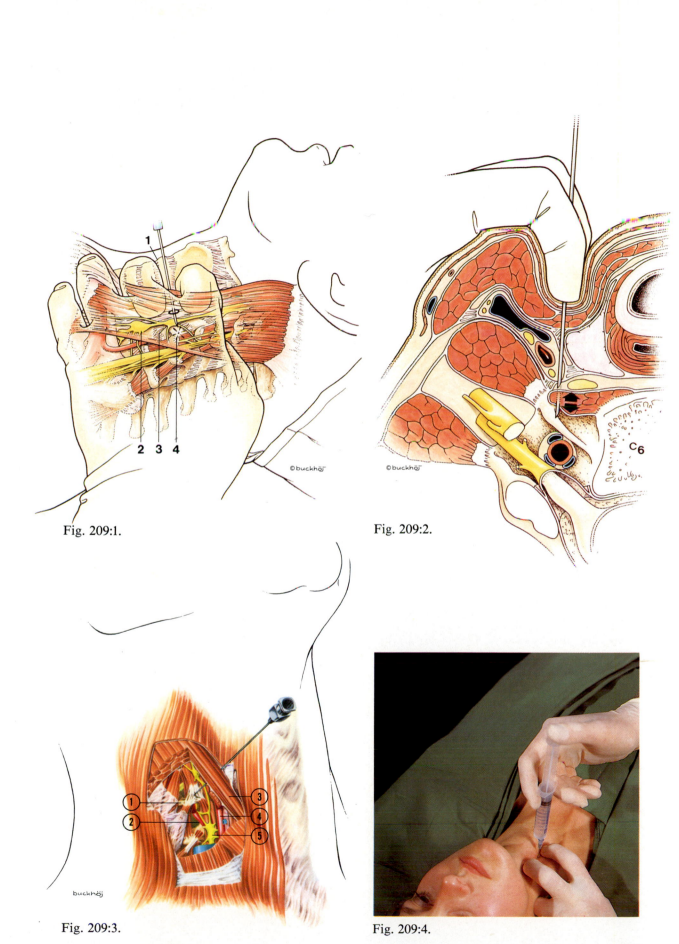

Fig. 209:1.

Fig. 209:2.

Fig. 209:3.

Fig. 209:4.

Coeliac plexus block

Anatomy
The coeliac plexus is situated retroperitoneally in the upper abdomen. It is at the level of the T12 and L1 vertebrae, anterior to the crura of the diaphragm. It surrounds the abdominal aorta and the coeliac and superior mesenteric arteries.

The plexus is composed of a network of nerve fibres, both sympathetic and parasympathetic. It contains two large coeliac ganglia, one on each side, which receive preganglionic sympathetic fibres from the three splanchnic nerves (greater, lesser and lowest). The plexus also receives parasympathetic fibres from the vagus nerve.

Connected to the coeliac plexus are numerous secondary plexuses such as the hepatic, gastric, splenic, renal, and suprarenal. From these are derived much of the autonomic supply to the abdominal viscera, including the kidneys and suprarenal glands, as well as to the blood vessels which supply them (Fig. 211:1).

Indications
1. Pain of acute or chronic pancreatitis.
2. Visceral pain due to cancer.
3. As an adjunct to intercostal, epidural or spinal anaesthesia for upper abdominal operations.

Patient position
Prone with pillow under abdomen.

Landmarks
1. Twelfth ribs
2. Spinous process of L2

Needle insertion
A 10-15 cm 18 or 20 gauge needle is used. A skin wheal is raised 8 cm lateral to the midline at the lower border of the 12th rib. This should be at the level of the L1 vertebra. The needle is inserted medially at 45° so as to miss the transverse spinous process and contact the body of the L1 vertebra. It is then withdrawn and reinserted a little steeper so as to glide past the vertebral body. After advancing slowly for 2-3 cm, the needle position should be checked radiologically. The tip should be 1-2 cm anterior to the vertebral body in a lateral view and within the lateral border of the body in an anteroposterior view (Figs. 211:2 and 211:3).

Because the aorta (left side) and the inferior vena cava (right side) are close to the coeliac plexus, a constant watch should be kept for blood escaping from the needle hub (Fig. 211:4).

The position of the needle is further confirmed by injecting 1-2 ml of radio-opaque dye using the image intensifier. The dye should remain close to the vertebral body. Intravascular or intraperitoneal injection will be readily identified.

Drugs and dose
If local anaesthetic is to be used, then 20 ml of 1% lidocaine or 0.25% bupivacaine or their equivalent should be injected. It is usual to inject the coelic plexus bilaterally although the injectate can cross the midline if enough is used. This can be checked radiologically if dye is added to the local anaesthetic.

If a neurolytic agent is to be used, then alcohol is the most frequently employed. Concentrations from 50-100% (20 ml per side, or 40 ml on one side if it is seen to spread bilaterally) have been recommended. Injected by itself, alcohol can be quite painful and with coeliac plexus block the patient may complain of a pain similar to a blow to the solar plexus. This pain can be prevented or largely modified by first injecting 5-10 ml of 1% lidocaine, and allowing up to 5 min before injecting the alcohol. It should contain some radio-opaque dye to check the position of the injectate.

Phenol 6-10% may also be used and has the advantage of being painless upon injection.

If being used as an adjunct for upper abdominal surgery it is clearly not practical to do a coeliac plexus block under radiological control before surgery in many operating theatres. If the block is to be used in abdominal surgery then an anterior approach under direct vision can be used. The viscera are retracted until the aorta can be palpated as it enters the abdomen. A needle is inserted close to one side of the aorta so as to contact the vertebra. 20-25 ml of 1% lidocaine or 0.25% bupivacaine is injected and the injection repeated on the opposite side of the aorta.

Complications

Entry of the needle tip into a large vessel, the peritoneal cavity or a viscus should all be diagnosed before injection if the procedure is done with radiological control.

1. Hypotension is sometimes seen, particularly orthostatic hypotension. This may last up to 3 days and should be treated with bed rest and avoidance of sudden changes to the upright posture.
2. Backache may be due to local trauma, irritation of alcohol in the psoas muscle or the involvement of the lumbar plexus.
3. Retroperitoneal haemorrhage.

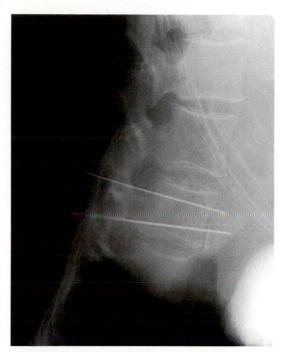

Figs. 211:2.
Needle points 1-2 cm in front of L1 and within the shadow of the lateral wall of the vertebral body. Courtesy of Dr. G.R.M. Carmichael.

Fig. 211:1.

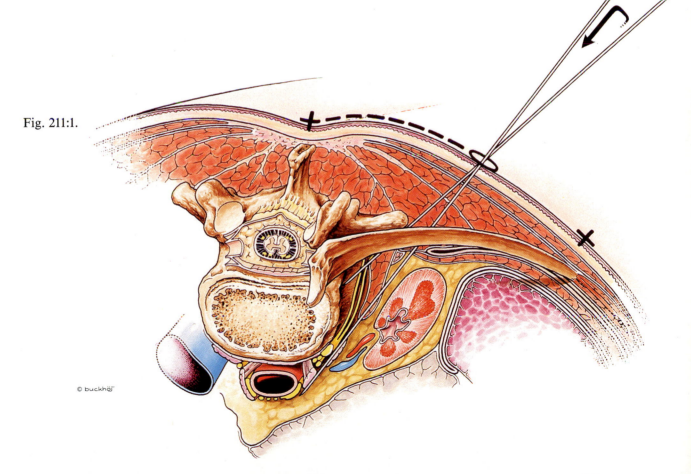

© buckhöj

Splanchnic nerve block

Because all the sympathetic sensory nerves from the abdominal viscera are located within the splanchnic nerves, it is possible to achieve the same analgesic results by blocking the splanchnic nerves as would be obtained with a coeliac plexus block. The parasympathetic nerves and many of the afferent sympathetic pathways involving the coeliac plexus remain undisturbed.

Anatomy

There are three splanchnic nerves, the greater, the lesser and the lowest. The **greater splanchnic nerve** is derived from sympathetic (afferent and efferent) fibres arising in or passing through the 5th to the 9th thoracic ganglia of the sympathetic chain. It runs over the bodies of the thoracic vertebra, becoming more anterior as it descends. It enters the abdomen by piercing the crus of the diaphragm and ends in the coeliac plexus. The **lesser splanchnic nerve** is from fibres arising in or passing through the 10th and 11th thoracic ganglia, and the **lowest splanchnic nerve** from the 12th ganglia. All three nerves are in close relationship with each other as they enter the abdomen on the anterior and superior aspect of the 12th thoracic vertebra (Fig. 213:1 and 2).

Indications

1. Pain of acute or chronic pancreatitis
2. Visceral pain due to cancer

Patient position

Prone with a pillow under the abdomen.

Landmarks

1. Twelfth rib
2. Midline

Needle insertion

A wheal is raised 8-10 cm lateral to the midline just below the 12th rib. The needle is inserted cephalad and medially so as to contact the body of the 12th thoracic vertebra (Fig. 213:4). Using radiological control the needle is redirected and advanced until it is over the upper and anterior quadrant of the body of the 12th vertebra in the lateral view and within the lateral boundaries of the vertebral body in the anteroposterior view (Fig. 213:3).

Drugs and dose

A preliminary injection of 1-2 ml of radio-opaque dye is made to exclude an intravascular position of the needle. If the dye stays in close relationship to the vertebral body, then 10 ml of 6-10% phenol with added dye may be injected.

If a local anaesthetic is to be used (e.g. in acute pancreatitis) then 10-15 ml of 1% lidocaine or 0.25% bupivacaine or their equivalent should be used and a catheter similar to that used for continuous epidural block can be inserted for repeated injections.

A bilateral injection may be necessary, but substantial pain relief can occur with a unilateral block. If a bilateral block is done then care must be taken in interpreting the lateral view of the radiological picture, and it is helpful to screen continuously during the injection.

Complications

Orthostatic hypotension.

Fig. 213:1.
1. Greater splanchnic nerve
2. Lesser splanchnic nerve
3. Least splanchnic nerve
4. Coeliac ganglion and plexus
5. Left branch of hepatic artery
6. Right branch of hepatic artery
7. Cystic artery
8. Common hepatic artery and hepatic plexus
9. Right gastric artery
10. Gastroduodenal artery
11. Superior pancreaticoduodenal artery
12. Right gastroepiploic artery
13. Superior mesenteric ganglion, artery and plexus
14. Aorticorenal ganglion and renal artery with plexus
15. Ovarian/testicular artery and plexus
16. Phrenic plexus and inferior phrenic artery
17. Left gastric artery and plexus
18. Splenic artery and plexus
19. Pancreatic branch
20. Gastric arteries
21. Splenic branch
22. Abdominal aortic plexus
23. Inferior mesenteric ganglion, artery and plexus
24. Superior hypogastric plexus
25. Inferior hypogastric plexus
26. Pelvic plexus
27. Pelvic splanchnic nerve (nervus erigens)
28. Pudendal nerve

Figs. 213:3. Courtesy of Dr. D.G. Littlewood

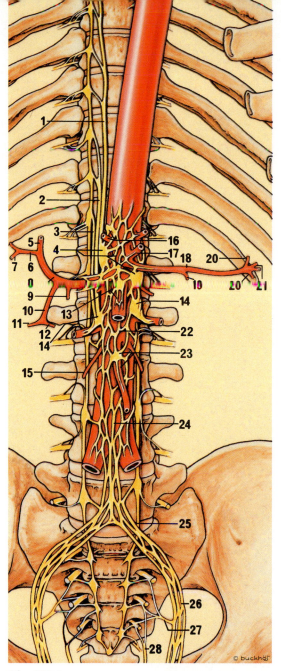

Fig. 213:1.

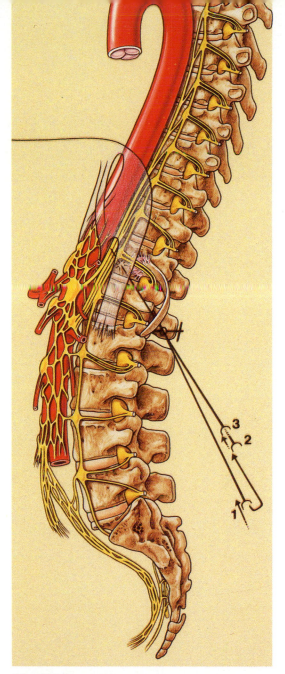

Fig. 213:2

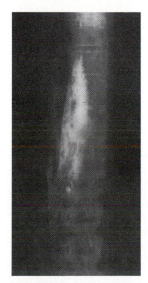

Fig. 213:3.

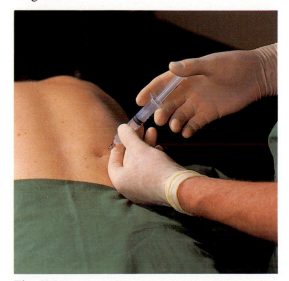

Fig. 213:4.

Suggested further reading

Boas, R.A. (1978). Sympathetic blocks in clinical practice. In Regional Anesthesia: Advances and selected topics, Vol. 16, International Anesthesia Clinics. Ed. Stanton-Hicks M. d'A. Little, Brown, Boston, p. 149.

Katz, J. and Renck, H. (1987). Handbook of Thoraco-abdominal Nerve Block. Mediglobe, Fribourg.

Löfström, J.B. and Cousins, M.C. (1988). Sympathetic neural blockade of upper and lower extremity. In Neural Blockade, eds Cousins, M.C. and Bridenbaugh, P.O. Lippincott, Philadelphia, p. 461.

Moore, D.C. (1975). Regional Block. C. C. Thomas Springfield, Illinois.

Postoperative pain relief

One of the main advantages of regional anaesthesia is that following surgery the residual nerve block gives excellent postoperative pain relief as long as the local anaesthetic drug maintains its effect. The duration of this residual block will of course be very variable, depending on the length of operation, the drug used and its dosage, the nerve block employed, etc. However, there are many ways in which the block may be extended to the patient's advantage.

The techniques do not have to be complicated, e.g. a ring block of the big toe will give many hours of comfort after removal of the toe-nail. Even when general anaesthesia has been used, a nerve block can greatly assist in providing analgesia after surgery.

It should not be expected that the regional anaesthesia will always give excellent analgesia by itself. While it may anaesthetise the wound, pain or discomfort outwith the operative site can still occur e.g. diaphragmatic pain or the presence of a nasogastric tube. However, the reduction in the total amount of pain achieved by the local anaesthetic greatly assists parenteral analgesic in achieving a high success rate. When using regional anaesthesia postoperatively, ensure that adequate amounts of analgesics are also prescribed.

Local infiltration

Wound infiltration
Subcutaneous infiltration of the wound by the surgeon just before skin closure can anaesthetise the skin for many hours. Bupivacaine 0.5% with or without epinephrine 1:200.000 will give several hours of skin anaesthesia. Methods using catheters implanted subcutaneously, and also in the muscle layers, have been used to allow further injections or a continuous infusion.

Ring block of digits
(See p. 114 and p. 140).

Arthroscopy
(See p. 40). Leaving a small quantity, e.g. 5-10 ml of 0.5% bupivacaine within the knee joint at the completion of arthroscopy will give good analgesia.

Minor nerve blocks

Iliohypogastric and ilioinguinal nerve blocks
(See p. 44). These blocks are easily performed and can be used for analgesia after herniorrhaphies.

Foot blocks
(See p. 134). Blockade of the tibial, the superficial and the deep peroneal nerves at the foot will provide analgesia after most foot operations, especially after hallux valgus operations.

Wrist blocks
(See p. 112). These blocks are simple to perform and useful after hand surgery.

Penile block
Penile block after operations such as circumcision is especially useful in children.

Terminal branches of the trigeminal nerves
(See p. 56). These nerves can be blocked after oral or facial surgery.

Major nerve blocks

Brachial plexus block
(See p. 90). This block is very useful after microsurgery of the hand as it not only provides analgesia but also maintains sympathetic blockade and consequent vasodilatation. A catheter such as an IV cannula can be implanted percutaneously within the neurovascular sheath and repeat injections are then possible.

Femoral nerve block
(See p. 122). This block will give excellent analgesia in patients with a fractured shaft of femur.

Intercostal nerve block
Blockade of the T6-T11 intercostal nerves gives good results after unilateral abdominal incisions, e.g. for cholecystectomy. Using 0.5% bupivacaine 6-12 h of analgesia can be obtained (see p. 144).

Cryoanalgesia of the intercostal nerves performed while the thorax is open has been used for pain relief after thoracotomy. Good relief is obtained particularly after the intercostal drain has been removed, but there have been reports of troublesome neuropathy.

Cryoanalgesia of the intercostal nerves performed while the thorax is open has been used for pain relief after thoracotomy. Good relief is obtained particularly after the intercostal drain has been removed, but there have been reports of troublesome neuropathy.

Interpleural injection
(See p. 150). This is particularly effective after subcostal (Kocher) incisions for cholecystectomy, but it has also been used for thoracotomy, fractured ribs, renal surgery and mastectomy.

Bupivacaine is the preferred drug. Several dosage regimes have been used and only seem to differ in regard to the duration of effect, the more local anaesthetic used, the longer being the duration. Thus 20 ml of 0.25% will last on average about 4 h, 20 ml 0.375% 6 h and 20 ml 0.5% 8 h. Individual variations are quite wide and top-ups should be given as required. The plasma concentrations that have been measured indicate a slow uptake from the pleural cavity and toxic levels are not seen. Epinephrine 1:200.000 is usually added to the solution.

To avoid top-up injections, continuous infusions have been used, e.g. 5-10 ml/h of 0.25% or 0.5% bupivacaine.

Central nerve blocks

Epidural block
Although the effectiveness of epidural block in relieving postoperative pain is undoubted and the use of a catheter technique allows for continuous use over many hours or days, this technique has not achieved the popularity in postoperative analgesia that it has with the relief of pain in labour.

Advantages
Nevertheless, excellent results can be obtained, and the following advantages may accrue from its use:
1. Excellent pain relief without central depression
2. Protection from the surgical stress reaction
3. Increase in lower limb blood flow with a decrease in the incidence of deep venous thrombosis and pulmonary embolus
4. Avoidance of postoperative hypertension, e.g. after major arterial surgery
5. Ability to passively move replaced joints and institute physiotherapy without pain
6. Better gastrointestinal function as the inhibitory effects of opioids can be avoided

Side-effects
The most feared side-effects are:

Hypotension
This is seldom a problem if patients are properly hydrated, the block is restricted to the segments required for analgesia, and sudden movement to the sitting up position is avoided. Arterial blood pressure is easy to monitor and hypotension is easy to treat, e.g. by giving IV fluids and/or a vasopressor.

Prolonged paralysis of the lower limbs
This is disliked by the patients but can be avoided by proper selection of the concentration of local anaesthetic.

Catheter migration to the subarachnoid space
This has been described but it must be extremely rare. Plastic catheters used in epidural blocks cannot be pushed through normal dura mater. Apparent migration can often be explained by the use of a multiple hole catheter which may have been inserted in such a way that the distal hole is within the subarachnoid space while the proximal holes are in the epidural space. In such an eventuality, a slow injection would deposit drug in the epidural space while a fast injection would force it into the subarachnoid space.

Urinary retention
This is common with epidural blocks that involve the sacral nerve roots containing the sacral parasympathetic nerves. It does necessitate catheterisation of the bladder and prophylactic antibiotic is a prudent precaution.

Principles

Unlike its use in surgical operations, when a widespread block is usually desirable, a continuous epidural block for postoperative pain should be confined to a few spinal segments related to the incision site. Thus the catheter should be placed close to the centre of the required band of analgesia and only a small volume of local anaesthetic need be used. However, the smaller the volume, and therefore the dose, the shorter the duration of effect. Thus to maintain the analgesia, top-up injections must be frequent (e.g. hourly) or a continuous infusion must be maintained. Specially controlled syringes can inject preset volumes at preset intervals. Excellent analgesia will be maintained if the top-ups are given before the previous injection has worn off. Small volume high concentration injections will give the best results.

Continuous infusions can be made with more conventional pumps that are available in most hospitals. The best results are obtained with high volume, low concentration infusions after an initial bolus of relatively concentrated local anaesthetic. A low concentration infusion can maintain a block but not induce one. Should the sensory block become insufficient, then a further bolus dose will be required.

Site of catheter

This depends upon the site of the operation and may be:

1. Cervical, for operations on the upper limb, particularly those involving microsurgery.
2. Thoracic for thoracotomies and abdominal surgery. Upper abdominal operations should have a catheter inserted to T8, while with lower abdominals it can be inserted at T11.
3. Lumbar for operations on the hips, knees and perineum.
4. Sacral for perineal operations.

Drugs and dose

Bupivacaine is the agent of choice as it causes less motor block than other drugs. In general midthoracic blocks require less volume than the other sites of injection. 4-5 ml can block several segments with such blocks, while lower thoracic or lumbar injections may need twice this volume for the initial injections.

If an epidural block has been used during the operation, then a top up, using 0.5% bupivacaine, should be made at the end of surgery. If repeated bolus injections are to be made, then the extent of the block 1h later should be determined and from this the volume of subsequent injections can be estimated.

If a continuous infusion is to be used, then this should be started as soon as the patient is in recovery. Dosage recommendations are given in Table 220:1. However, the extent of the block should be checked 3-4 h after the initial top-up (or if the patient complains of pain) to see if it is optimal. If not the rate of infusion can be adjusted, remembering that if there is an inadequate band of anaesthesia, a bolus injection will be required as well as an increase in the infusion rate.

Monitoring

The following should be monitored and recorded:

1. Heart rate and arterial pressure. Initially these should be measured fairly frequently, but once the patient is stabilised, hourly recordings are sufficient. If a bolus injection is given then recordings should be made every 5 min for 15 min.

2. The amount of drug infused every hour.

3. The height and intensity of the block. Nurses can be taught to estimate the upper extent of the sensory block (e.g. using a piece of ice) and the degree of motor block (e.g. by asking the patient to move the lower limbs).

A special form for the nursing staff indicating the variables to be monitored, the prescribed dose to be infused and instructions on the management of hypotension is particularly valuable for managing these patients. Simple measures to counteract hypotension such as raising the foot of the bed, giving 250-500 ml of IV electrolyte solution quickly or injecting ephedrine 20-30 mg intramuscularly, should be taught to the nursing staff. An anaesthetist should always be present in the hospital for consultation and action.

Concomitant analgesics

As mentioned at the beginning of this chapter, complete analgesia of the operation wound may not be enough to make the patient completely comfortable. Other parenteral analgesics, particularly opioids, will usually be required and should not be withheld. Apart from dealing with pain or discomfort outwith the blocked area, they will often provide much needed sedation. Conventional doses given by the intramuscular route, e.g. 10 mg morphine, will have particularly good analgesic effect when the main postoperative pain has been relieved by the epidural block.

Epidural opioids

It is well established that opioids injected into the epidural space can cross the dura mater and gain access to the dorsal horns of the spinal cord. By attaching themselves to μ-receptors in the substantia gelatinosa of the dorsal horns, they produce excellent analgesia without obvious neural blockade. The doses required are generally less than is used intramuscularly, but there is a wide individual variation in regard to effectiveness and duration.

The oil/water partition coefficient of the various opioids is very important. Low lipid solubility increases the time required for the drug to reach the spinal cord, but increases the duration of effect as the drug will leave the cord only slowly. However, the relatively high water solubility of such drugs will lead to high concentrations in the cerebrospinal fluid and the possibility of cephalad migration with consequent respiratory depression. Morphine, which is the most commonly used drug for this purpose, has a low partition coefficient. Its onset time is long, but its duration is also long, hence its popularity. However, it has been responsible for the great majority of respiratory depressions that have been reported, the incidence of cases requiring active treatment of the depression being of the order of 1 in 200.

High lipid solubility on the other hand leads to a shorter onset and a low incidence of respiratory depression, but the duration is relatively short. Drugs such as fentanyl (and its derivatives), pethidine, methadone and diamorphine all have high lipid solubility and if used alone required frequent injections. Lipid soluble drugs should be injected at or near the appropriate spinal segments subserving the pain, as they will occupy receptors in the nearest part of the spinal cord and be unable to migrate any distance.

Most opioids are given epidurally in doses 20-50% of that usually used IM.

Complications

The main side effects are:

1. Respiratory depression. This unfortunately is not easy to monitor though the respiratory rate may be helpful. Particular care is necessary if IM opioid has also been given.
2. Pruritis. Usually this is tolerable but can be troublesome.
3. Urinary retention.
4. Nausea and vomiting.

Naloxone is effective in reversing respiratory depression but it may have to be continued for many hours. It will also reverse excessive pruritis without affecting the analgesia.

Combination of local anaesthetic drugs and opioids

Several studies have now shown that the best results in treating postoperative pain come from epidural injections of a mixture of a local anaesthetic and an opioid, particularly when given as an infusion.

Because the two drugs have a different site of action, the dose of each can be kept to a minimum with a consequent reduction in side-effects.

Because the duration of effect of a drug is of little consequence when given by continuous infusion, it is possible to use an opioid of high lipid solubility with little risk of respiratory depression, e.g. fentanyl, sufentanyl or diamorphine, given at 5-10% of their normal IM dose per hour, mixed with 0.125% bupivacaine at 15 ml/h. Morphine at a rate of 0.5 mg/h is also effective mixed with 0.125% bupivacaine. The avoidance of bolus doses of opioid may also protect against respiratory depression.

The local anaesthetic drug will retain most of the advantages of continuous nerve block mentioned above.

Suggested regimes
See Tables 220:1 and 220:2.

Table 220:1.

Operation site	Catheter position	Initial bolus dose Bupi- vacaine 0.5%	Infusion rate Bupivacaine 0.125%
Thoracic and upper abdominal	T6-T8	4-6 ml	5-10 ml/h
Lower abdominal	T10	10 ml	15 ml/h
Hip or knee replacement	L2-3	8 ml	10 ml/h

The initial bolus dose should be given at the end of surgery and the infusion started soon thereafter. If the block wears off, another bolus of 0.5% bupivacaine should be given and the infusion rate increased.

Table 220:2.

Morphine	0.5 mg/h
Diamorphine	0.5 mg/h
Pethidine	10 mg/h
Fentanyl	10 ug/h
Alfentanil	50 ug/h

Recommended infusion rate of opioids if added to 0.125% bupivacaine. The opioid is added direct to the bupivacaine, the dose depending on the rate of infusion - see Table 220:1.

Spinal anaesthesia (see p. 194)

Continuous spinal anaesthesia using a catheter technique is gaining in popularity. Although it can involve piercing the dura with an 18 gauge needle, the incidence of spinal headache is surprisingly low, possibly due to the fact that most patients are elderly.

The advantage of the technique is that only very small quantities of local anaesthetic are required for each injection, eliminating unusually high blocks and the danger of toxicity.

Until there are further data on continuous infusions, the method of choice is repeated bolus injection. The amount given, the baricity of the solution and the position of the patient will be determined by the site of operation and the ability to position the patient appropriately. Thus following a hip operation, a patient who is sitting up may be given 0.75-1.5 ml of hyperbaric solution, while one who is nursed horizontal would do better with 0.75-1.5 ml of isobaric or hypobaric solution. The extent and effectiveness of the block should be determined 20-30 min after the initial injection and appropriate modification to the dose made if necessary. Full aseptic precautions must be taken, particularly the use of a bacterial filter attached to the catheter.

Spinal opioids

Opioids injected into the cerebrospinal fluid are much more rapid in their onset than those used epidurally, and the dose required is about 10-20% of the epidural dose. The incidence of respiratory depression is much higher than with epidural administration and the method cannot be recommended outside intensive care units. Even in such units the possibility of late respiratory depression and apnoea requires constant vigilance.

Conclusion

Much more could be done for patient comfort after operation if regional anaesthetic technique were more widely used, even with operations performed under general anaesthesia. Many of these techniques can be quickly and easily performed and pose little or no risk to the patient. The more complex methods require more dedication and particularly the co-operation and enthusiasm of an informed nursing staff.

Suggested further reading

Scott D.B. (1988). Management of acute pain. In Neural Blockade, eds. Cousins, M.C. and Bridenbaugh, P.O. Lippincott, Philadelphia, p. 861.

Index